RAW FOOD
real world

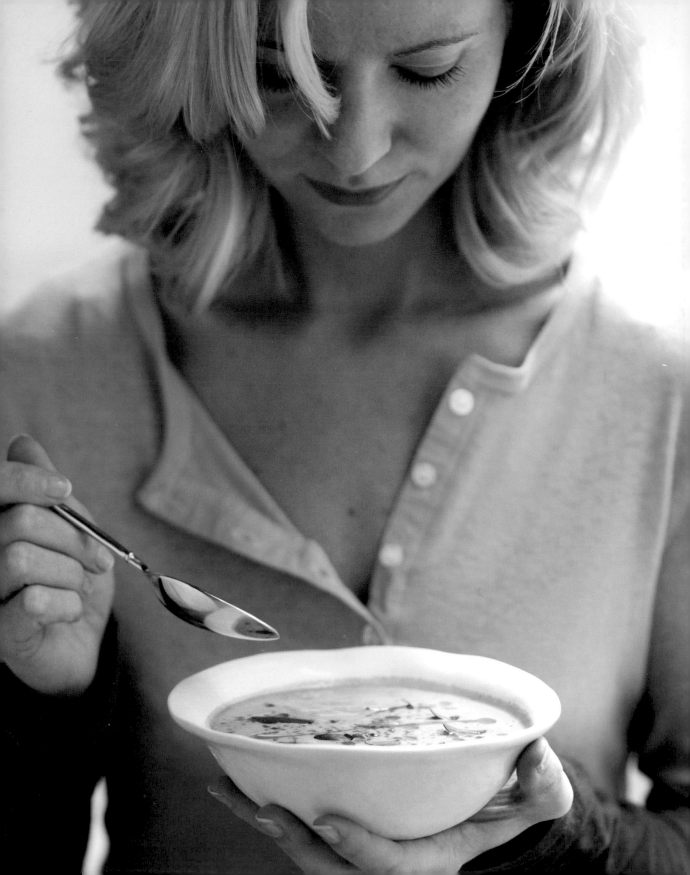

RAW FOOD
real world
100 RECIPES TO GET THE GLOW

MATTHEW KENNEY AND
SARMA MELNGAILIS

WITH JEN KARETNICK

10 ReganBooks
Celebrating Ten Bestselling Years
An Imprint of HarperCollinsPublishers

HarperCollins books may be purchased for educational, business, or sales promotional use. For information please write: Special Markets Department, HarperCollins Publishers Inc., 10 East 53rd Street, New York, NY 10022.

FIRST EDITION

Art Direction and Design by Michelle Ishay

All photographs by Charles Schiller except for pages 10, 13, 14, 190, 249, 255, 275, 292, 356 by John Botte and page 33 by Carina Salvi.

Printed on acid-free paper

Library of Congress Cataloging-in-Publication Data

Kenney, Matthew.
    Raw food/real world : 100 recipes to get the glow / Matthew Kenney and Sarma Melngailis.
    — 1st ed.
        p.   cm.
    ISBN 0-06-079355-4
    1. Vegetarian cookery. 2. Raw foods. I. Melngailis, Sarma, 1972– II. Title.

05 06 07 08 09 RRD 10 9 8 7 6 5 4 3 2 1

To Matthew

—S.M.

To Sarma

—M.K.

To Jon, Zoe, and Remy,
with love and mangos

—J.K.

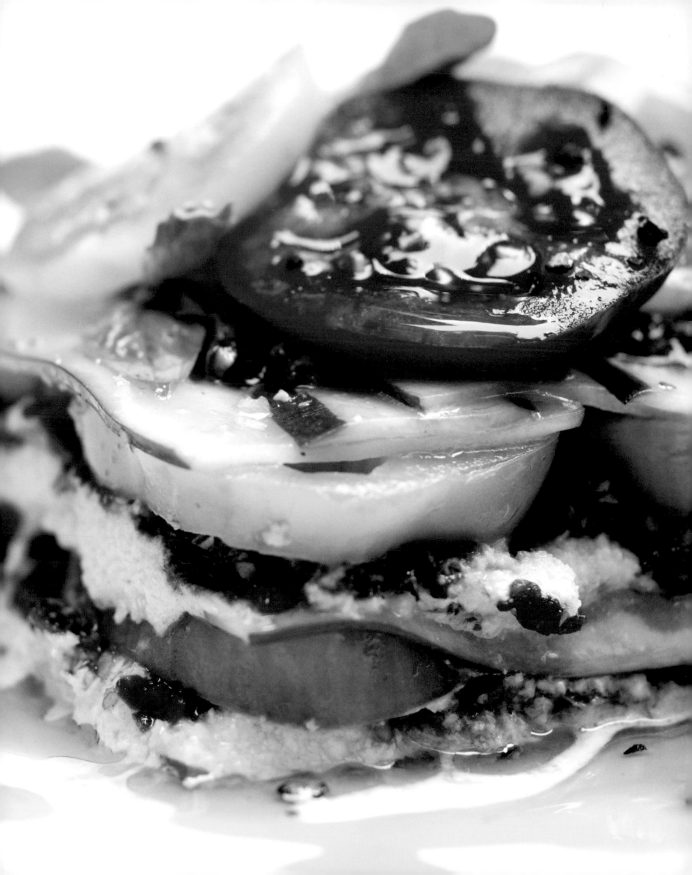

CONTENTS

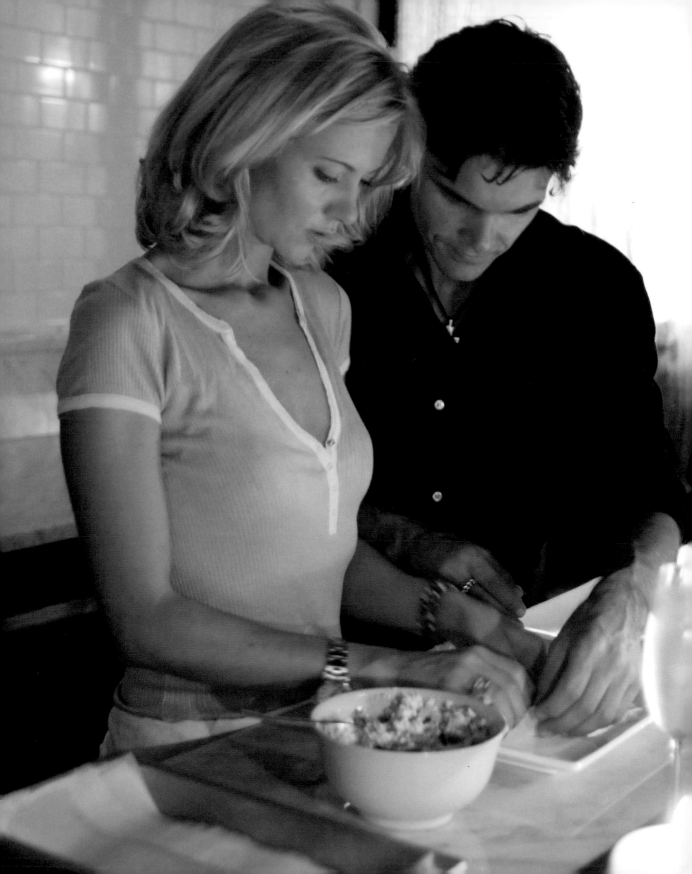

INTRODUCTION
GET THE GLOW

It sounds like a promise made in an advertisement for a luxurious beauty cream—buy this and you, too, can have this fabulous glow —something just a little too good be true. But for those who live the raw food lifestyle and invest as much thought into the process as into the product, it's too true not to be good.

People who eat only raw, plant-based foods have an unmistakable shine, like a pregnant woman in her second trimester or someone newly in love. They have a radiant, positive energy. It's easy to spot a raw foodist in a crowd of people living on the Standard American Diet (SAD . . . an appropriate acronym!). Just look for unusually clear skin, glossy hair, and shining eyes.

When you cook foods, the colors and textures change and all the precious water is burned off. Eating raw food keeps you closer to the earth and connects you to the original product, the real thing. Think about biting into a perfectly sun-ripened peach just plucked from a tree. This is the ideal way to eat—sensual, sexy, and energizing. If we just served fruits and vegetables on plates, of course, we would not have much of a restaurant or a book, nor any outlet to do what we love: preparing food that is creative, exciting, and satisfying. We may blend, chop, and even dehydrate, but still the integrity of the product, specifically the nutrients and enzymes, remain intact. Eating food that is alive keeps you feeling alive.

But more profoundly, living on raw foods enables you to effortlessly shed not only excess physical weight; other, less tangible burdens are lifted. For some, it's that overall "unhealthy relationship" with food. For others, it's the persistent and lingering fear of disease which we can begin to let go of with the reassurance of knowing that good health is our natural right and we are now armed to claim it. Further, there can be an indescribable happiness, along with the sense of communion, that comes from not eating animals anymore, being less taxing to the environment, and reducing the weight upon the medical community—in short, living in a way that lessens the burden on the rest of the world.

But before you slam this book shut and head for the nearest burger counter, keep in mind that our own transition to raw foods had nothing at all to do with animal rights or the environment. It was simply about wanting to feel our best physically. We had no idea about the bonuses that would come along with it, in particular the incredible increase in overall energy, somehow also accompanied by a greater sense of peace.

In this book we share our story, our advice, and our recipes in what we hope is a practical and accessible way. Our introduction to the world of raw foods was a sudden one. While we both felt like we'd stumbled onto something extraordinary, it was not always a smooth ride. We are both classically trained chefs with a shared love of restaurants and good food. Then literally overnight, we went from cooking and eating all varieties of meat, fish, and fowl, plus dairy, sugar, flour, and everything in between, to working with and consuming only *raw plant foods*—and we did this without really knowing what we were doing or what to expect. We just recognized that we wanted to do it and that it felt right. We also happened to discover raw foods when we had the luxury of a great deal of free time, and so dove into it full force by reading and researching, attending seminars, participating in grueling and complicated cleanses, and getting to know the still predominantly underground world of raw foods. Some of these experiences were more than a little colorful, but throughout, we learned how ordinary people with regular jobs and social lives can incorporate raw foods into their daily routines in a meaningful, practical, and delicious way.

In short, it is our bold claim that raw foods can change your life. A raw food diet is not a trend, a tool, a religion, or some kind of cult. It doesn't have to be all about sacrifice or discipline. You can incorporate raw foods into your own lifestyle to whatever degree, at whatever pace you wish. Just be prepared to feel happier, sexier, more vibrant, energetic, and at peace with yourself and the rest of the world, even if that isn't your intention. And, of course, be ready to exercise your right to glow.

What Is Raw Food?

The raw food "movement," a plant-based, vegan lifestyle, has been around for a long time. It has a bunch of other nicknames—live food, living cuisine, sunfood cuisine—and there are slight distinctions, though the polemics spring from the same essential source. But no matter the label, the connotation is the same: It is a diet comprising naturally grown wild or organically and sustainably raised fruits, vegetables, nuts, seeds, and occasionally sprouted grains. Like vegans, raw foodists do not consume animal products of any kind (with the exception, in many cases, of honey and bee pollen). However, the raw food lifestyle goes further by excluding any foods with chemically processed or pasteurized ingredients. Finally, and most significantly, during the preparation of raw food dishes, nothing is cooked, at least in the traditional sense.

This may sound limiting to some. But for us, the possibilities that exist within the raw food lifestyle are both boundless and thoroughly satisfying. When you are able to enjoy a simple bowl of sweet cherries, or a creamy avocado with a splash of lime juice and coarse sea salt, it is easy to imagine how a little creativity can make this food exciting. In fact, raw food has its own cuisine identity, and it is very much a playful and inventive one. But the real benefit of raw food, aside from great flavor, is the unbelievable way it makes you feel, inside and out.

OUR STORY

MK: "I was raised on the coast of Maine, surrounded by fresh, seasonal foods, which became the foundation for the standards I have now developed. When I first moved to New York, I very quickly became fascinated and literally fell in love with restaurants. I started out waiting tables at a Sicilian restaurant, and then worked my way into the kitchen. The food at that restaurant exploded with flavor. I began to love the light yet intense Mediterranean way of cooking—the flavors of citrus, olive oil, seasonal fruits and vegetables, tons of fresh herbs and spices. I soon became aware, however, that I would need more than just restaurant experience, and I enrolled in culinary school.

When I finally had the opportunity to open my first restaurant, it was Mediterranean. In fact, the next four restaurants I opened after that were also Mediterranean. I traveled all over the world and brought influences from those travels into my kitchens. Although the restaurants I had opened were very well reviewed and did quite well, they did not have the critical mass that would be required to sustain them. Following a trend that was picking up in those days, my new partners and I began to shift the direction of my company toward American regional food, with an emphasis on heavier comfort foods. My heart was not in this in the least. My most successful restaurant was known for its Truffled Macaroni and Cheese, yet no one can ever claim to have seen me eat the dish, ever, because I never did. I didn't particularly enjoy that kind of food and did not like the way eating it made me feel. Nevertheless, the comfort food craze was lucrative and the restaurant business became just that to me, a business—no longer a passion."

SM: "I grew up in a suburb of Boston, Massachusetts, in a family where food was always very important. My mother was a professional chef who taught me a great deal and instilled in me a passion for food and cooking. After college, however, I moved to New York City to work in investment banking. It was only after six rather grueling years in finance that I finally gave in and left to attend culinary school."

MK: "I had just secured a second cookbook deal, focusing on the 'urban' foods that my new restaurants served. The working name was *Big City Cooking* (and it stuck). I was very busy, operating several businesses and a large catering company, and I needed to hire a recipe tester to work with me on developing and testing the dishes. My agent called and told me about someone who had recently graduated from the French Culinary Institute and who was a big fan of my first book, *Matthew Kenney's Mediterranean Cooking*.

"Sarma arrived at my office one morning for our interview, very casual, friendly, eager, knowledgeable, and organized. I hired her on the spot. Working on this book together wound up being far more interesting than I had originally anticipated. In addition to the heavier macaroni-and-cheese type dishes, the recipes also included many dishes that we envisioned together and some that Sarma created herself. These dishes were colorful, fresh, and vibrant, and were more reflective of the lighter way we both preferred to eat. In the end, the book was beautiful, and we also realized that we had a stronger connection with each other than just food. Over the course of that year, our own relationship ultimately developed. We found ourselves becoming partners at work and at home, moving in together with Sarma's two cats."

SM: "After cooking school, when the opportunity to work with Matthew suddenly presented itself, it felt like an eerily fortunate coincidence. I had only met him twice before, very briefly. I remember clearly the day I came across his first book in a store, bought it and read it at home, cover to cover. Little did I know then that only a few years later we would be working on a book, living together, and then opening restaurants—all in the first year of our relationship. That first restaurant reflected very much the food of *Big City Cooking*. It was a mix of hearty, comforting foods and lighter, vibrant dishes. I loved working in the kitchen and I loved the food. However, despite good reviews and a busy opening, that restaurant was built at a precarious time for Matthew's company overall and, along with his other restaurants, it was ultimately not able to withstand the difficult circumstances for New York City that began in the fall of 2001."

MK: "In the middle of my thirty-eighth year in 2002, the business I had built, with over 600 employees, essentially collapsed, leaving me with the loss of seven restaurants and an enormous mess to clean up. After several years of incredibly hard work, I was not only going to be starting over, but doing so while saddled with countless legal and financial problems. At the same time, my always-resilient body and mind were beginning to feel a bit tired—nothing drastic at first, but the change was approaching rapidly. Still, I attributed it to that stress-related, difficult time as well as simply growing older.

"I remember feeling that aging is a natural and unavoidable part of our lives— to be embraced and not resisted. I accepted each new ache and pain as an unavoidable additional step away from a vibrant youth. However, it all seemed to be accelerating. My hips, after years of long distance running, were developing arthritis when just a year earlier, I could easily go out and run ten miles without any pain. Suddenly walking to the post office was giving me a bit of trouble. My fingers were stiff in the morning; my knees were acting up a bit; my hair was not as thick or soft as it had been. Most interesting about all of this was that I just accepted it. Overall, I thought I still felt pretty good and looked very healthy—all on a relative basis, of course."

SM: "Looking back, I find it interesting that it was during this period of recuperation—with no restaurants open and only a consulting project here and there keeping us busy—that we came across raw foods. We must have been subconsciously ready. Our friend Robb was going to take us to dinner at a restaurant I had chosen, Jean-George Vongerichten's then-new Tribeca restaurant, 66. He called earlier that same day and explained that he had been eating differently for some time and would really feel more comfortable if he could take us to a 'raw' restaurant. Of course we said we didn't mind, but selfishly I was *very* unhappy. I had really been looking forward to this dinner at a brand-new, sleekly designed, much-hyped restaurant featuring one of Manhattan's best chefs. But instead, after doing a little research on the Internet, we resigned ourselves to a tedious evening in a weird place, eating strange and unappealing food.

The restaurant was tiny and the service painfully slow. It was a hot summer evening and their air conditioner was not working. Robb ordered everything for us, as he knew the menu well. Of course, much of our conversation ended up being about raw food. As Robb explained to us the basics of the philosophy, the food slowly arrived, one dish at a time, and it was *good*. The longer we sat and ate—and listened—the more intrigued we became. The tiny space filled up and there were people waiting for tables. A tall and radiant model came in to pick up her to-go order. A girl at the table beside us, eating alone, told us how much better she felt since eating only raw foods, but she said she wished there were more options available—a 'cool' place where she could take her friends. If we had been in a cartoon, this would have been the moment that a light bulb appeared over my head and Matthew's at the same time."

MK: "Being in the food business and a restaurant enthusiast, it was very rare for me to dine out and not have three courses and lots of wine and leave fully satisfied, a term that I now equate with being stuffed, bloated, tired, and uncomfortable. 'Satisfied' now means something entirely different to me—that my body has what it needs for maximum efficiency and minimal digestive effort. But on that particular night, Sarma and I were both struck by how alert, open-minded, energetic, and very, very clear we felt. It didn't take long before we realized this was something we needed to explore and try for ourselves."

SM: "We came up to our little summertime cottage in Maine, armed with books about raw food and a resolve to try eating only raw foods for two weeks. We were completely intrigued with raw food as a restaurant concept, and thought only that we should at least understand how it feels to eat raw food exclusively for a short time. We really thought it would be an interesting *experiment*. On the eve of our trial period, we sat down for one of our favorite summertime dinners, steamed lobsters. It was to be our last lobster dinner for a while, although neither of us had any clue at that time that it would really be our *last* lobster dinner.

"On our first days eating only raw food, we had plenty of fruit for breakfast. I made shakes in our blender with oranges, mangos, and pineapple. We ate lots of melon. We made huge salads and ate them out on the dock, reading books about raw food. We both became more and more engrossed.

"I felt great. We were not going to the gym or getting much exercise, but I somehow would wake every morning feeling so much better in my skin. I also slept like a baby, night after night. Before then, sleeping was a big issue for me. I didn't dare travel anywhere without my prescription of sleeping pills, but now I no longer needed them."

MK: "The most remarkable thing during our first go at raw food was that we did not crave other foods. In the past, we thought that we craved red meat or chicken or fish. We'd eat red meat at least once a week, feeling we needed it. Now we were not eating any animal foods at all, and had *no* cravings for it whatsoever. Nor did we crave dairy or sugar or bread. These initial stages of eating raw food were, however, a little challenging for me in other ways. My body did take time to adjust. Working out was a distant thought. I actually exercised less in the first few months of raw food than I had in the past twenty years. However, already quite lean, my weight began to drop. Meanwhile, I would go back and forth between feeling weak and tired and feeling like I'd discovered the fountain of youth."

SM: "I remember well the moment that I realized this was it—there was no going back. I was on the porch, reading a book about raw foods with my yellow marker in hand, furiously highlighting more of the text than not. I was reading a part about how humans are not biologically built to eat and digest meats and it was all making perfect, logical sense to me, and I wondered why I had never read this sort of information anywhere before. I put the book down, stared out at the ocean and considered for a moment—did I just become . . . a *vegan*?! It was exciting but also a bit scary at the same time. How would I tell my family? Did Matthew feel the same way? How would we break the news to foodie friends, who would surely make fun of us? How would we ever go *out* to dinner again? It was a bit sad, because cooking is an art based on years and years of tradition and history all built around family and celebrations, and now we were in a sense rejecting a large part of that history. And my lovely, shiny All Clad copper pots and Le Creuset baking dishes would now have no purpose but to collect dust. Still, despite the nostalgia of cooking and my fixation on the aesthetics of kitchenware, I was filled with such a profound happiness and excitement."

MK: "Fast-forward six months later: I was sitting on a plane, ready to take off for Maine, for my fifteenth college reunion. I felt an overwhelming energy, almost like a constant buzz, throughout my body and my mind was crystal clear. That was my first very profound recollection of how raw foods can and did make me feel—it is an incredible high, giving you strength, resolve, energy, and almost endless freedom from the constraints so often placed on us by our bodies. I had also reversed the weight loss that had made me look too skinny, and I felt stronger than ever.

"On the campus, I ran seven miles each day. My aches and pains were a distant memory, my eyes were becoming clear, my hair was thick and healthy, and my skin was starting to glow. Throughout the winter, surrounded by friends and coworkers who were ill, Sarma and I retained perfect health. We slept well, were making progress in every facet of our lives, and felt extremely happy with our revised outlook on our health and food."

SM: "Reading about how raw foods could change the way I felt was one thing, but experiencing it was quite another. Whereas Matthew seemed to need a little time to adjust, I felt dramatically better almost overnight. I also immediately noticed just feeling *better* in my skin. Today, the quality of my sleep has improved such that I feel great sleeping much *less*. My skin looks better, my eyes are clear, and things that used to stress me out or make me cranky seem to roll right off my back so much more easily."

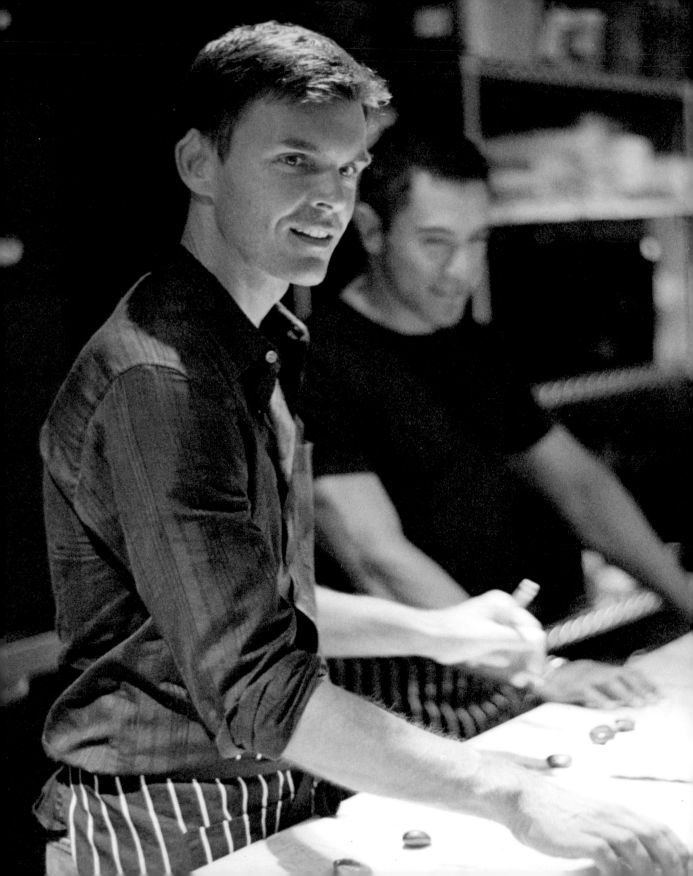

MK: "Going raw did (and still does today) present a philosophical dilemma for me. As a chef, I worked for years to build a career around the food that I created. Although I do not now embrace much of that kind of food as part of my own life, I respect it as an art form. The priorities in our lives have shifted, to the point where we still care very much about flavor and interesting food, but we are also equally concerned about what the food we put into our bodies does, in both the short and long term. If I had known then what I do now, I would have made the change twenty years ago."

SM: "What I love about this lifestyle is that anyone can start incorporating it into their own lives anytime and to whatever degree, and start to feel *better*. It does not require an immediate and complete overhaul—just an increasing awareness of how what you eat makes you feel and of adding more and more raw foods in place of others. I never really thought so much before about that old saying, 'you are what you eat', but it's true! Heavy and processed foods make you feel heavy and sluggish. Light, clean, natural, and alive foods make you feel light, clear, and more alive. And sexy. Take my word for it.

"I feel like I have a very clear understanding now of what my body needs and craves—some days I eat very little, some days much more. At times I can't get enough salad, wanting to eat bowlful after bowlful, while other days I'm not that interested and eat more fruit or I'll have some of the more complex dishes from our restaurant. I honestly don't crave processed sugary foods *ever*. What I do crave from time to time is raw cookies and ice creams, and I love that I can eat those whenever I want and not gain weight. All of the anxiety and guilt I used to associate with eating is gone, so in addition to being lighter physically, I feel lighter emotionally. I feel like I'm going through life now with a little happiness buzz."

MK: "The restaurant we opened in the summer of 2004, Pure Food and Wine, is unlike all of the other restaurants I have opened. It's not simply because there are no ovens, burners, fryers, or grills in the kitchen, but because it's truly the most personal expression of anything we have ever done. We even designed the space ourselves, feeling strongly that we would surely sacrifice some warmth and character if we hired a professional to do it for us. Our staff is passionate about what they do and we are lucky to be able to work with them all."

"Our goal was to create a comfortable, sexy, and inviting space that would attract not simply raw foodists, vegans, or vegetarians, but anyone who is interested in eating vibrant and flavorful food, perhaps trying something new, and feeling great. The response we most often get from first-time diners and people who are new to raw foods is that they are truly surprised at how satisfying and filling it can be, and by how good they feel at the end of the meal.

"Many of our regular customers, and in fact the majority of our guests on any given night, are not vegetarians. Of these, many are interested in raw foods, but most simply enjoy the experience for what it is. Still, we meet countless numbers of people every week who are interested in raw foods, but are intimidated by their lack of knowledge about how to prepare them within their everyday lifestyle. This is a legitimate concern, but not because raw food is so challenging. With proper planning and preparation, it can be very easy, and we've included recipes that are quick and simple as well as others that are more elaborate but certainly worth the effort if you choose to make them. This is a book about much more than just recipes, it's also about a philosophy of sorts, and about sharing information that we found very compelling in doing our own research. We have also included our thoughts and advice on this lifestyle and revealed some of our own experiences and adventures in exploring and transitioning to raw foods. And finally, like our restaurant, it's a very personal and honest expression that we hope will be at best inspiring and at least entertaining!"

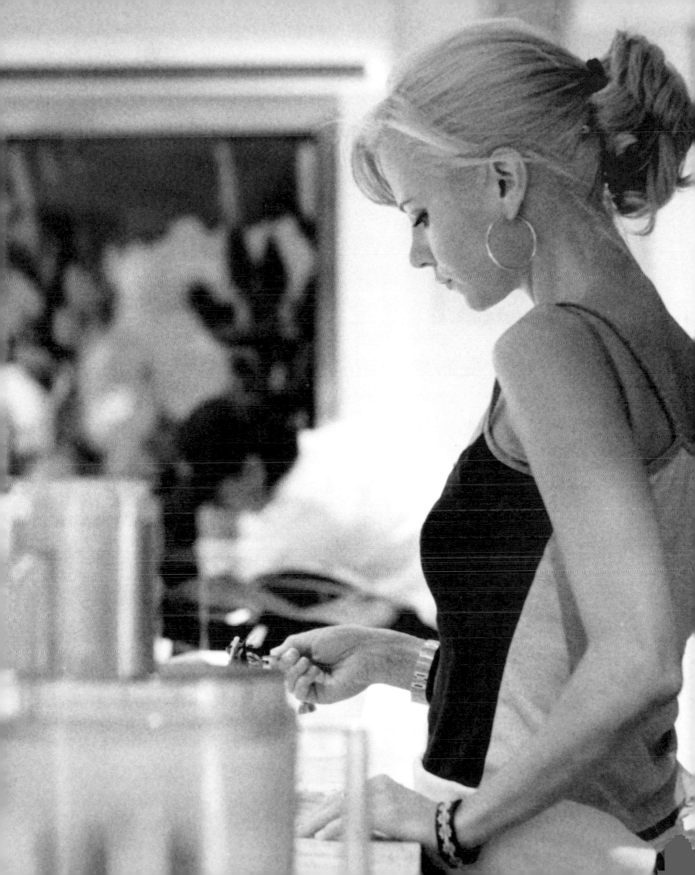

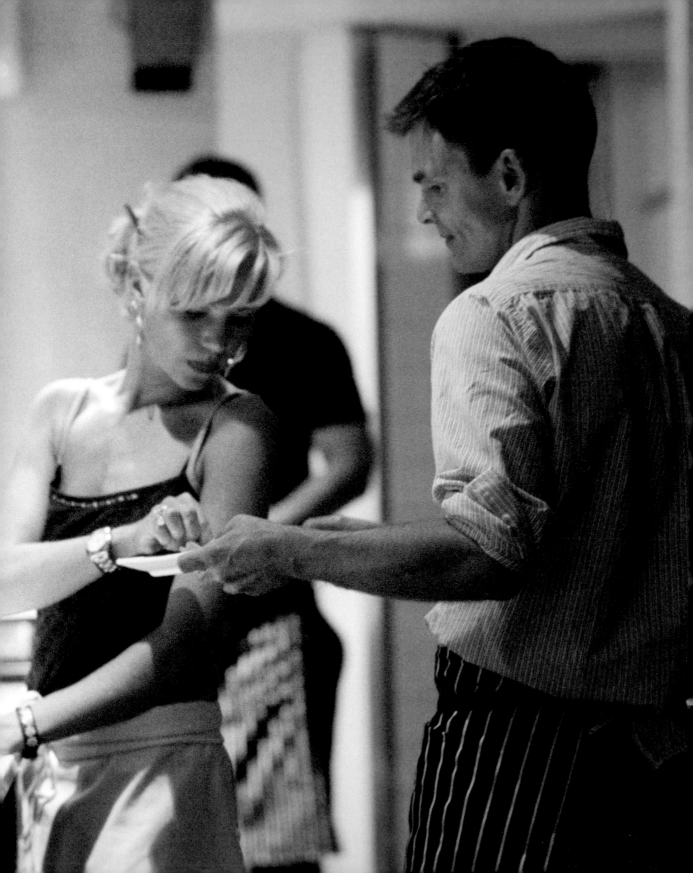

WHY WE GAVE UP COOKED FOOD AND MEAT

Given our shared passion for cooking, how is it that we were suddenly convinced to retire our pots and pans for good? It's not just the extra cupboard space that our oven now provides. It was the research. When we first began eating raw foods, we immediately dove into the history and rationale behind this way of eating. What we found not only explained the positive changes in the way we felt, but actually inspired a rather firm resolve to avoid cooked foods, meat, and dairy forever.

What's Not to Love About Cooked Food?

Raw foods contain live enzymes that aid in digestion, which activate as they are consumed. Heating foods to temperatures beyond 118°F causes those enzymes to begin to die, destroys nutrients and vitamins, and alters the natural metabolic structure of the food. Essentially, eating cooked food is an inefficient and ultimately deleterious way of feeding ourselves. Because the foods' enzymes have been destroyed, your body has to use or produce its own enzymes to digest the cooked food. As we age, our bodies' natural source of enzymes is depleted, and many believe that eating cooked food only hastens this process. As Dr. Gabriel Cousens, author of several books on raw foods, explains, "As our enzyme pool diminishes with age, our ability to perform the tasks that keep the body healthy also diminishes. Aging happens when enzymes decrease in concentration in the body." Therefore, Cousens continues, some enzyme researchers, like Dr. Edward Howell, the progenitor in this field, and live-food teachers like Ann Wigmore, believe that enzyme preservation is a secret to longevity. By eating raw foods, we build up our enzyme reserves.

> **The most significant change for me? I used to feel that every day I was growing older. Now I feel like every day I'm getting younger.** —MK

Furthermore, cooking food depletes and destroys vitamins, minerals, and amino acids. Deranged molecules in the food can break down into new and unnatural substances. This generates toxic substances, particularly in grilling or frying, many of which are carcinogenic. Cooking the water out of foods leaves behind only inferior fiber that has lost most of its intestine-cleansing properties. When we eat these nutrient-depleted foods, our bodies are still "hungry" for more food, because we need more nutrients that we can assimilate. Just as you wouldn't pour sludge into the tank of your new sports car along with gasoline, you can't fill your body with inferior fuel and expect it to function properly. To read more about the effects of cooking on food, check out Dr. Joseph Mercola's website, www.mercola.com, and type "raw food" into the search box.

Eating only raw plant foods is entirely amazing. It can give you so much energy; it's like a natural version of Ecstasy, and you never crash. —SM

Digesting raw foods simply does not consume our energy the same way that digesting cooked foods does. Think about that "food coma" you get after eating a big, heavy meal, or the post-lunchtime yearning for a nap. These symptoms and inappropriate or untimely desires will disappear. When you eat raw foods, you are eating clean foods that are easy to digest and that don't sap your energy. Having clean "pipes" also allows foods to pass through your body more quickly and efficiently!

How liberating not to have to scrub and scrape greasy pots and pans anymore. Think about how all that cooked grease so stubbornly sticks to the pans. What does it do to the inside of your body? —SM

Humans, domesticated pets, and farm animals are the only species that eat cooked food. They are also the only ones that get degenerative diseases. You don't see wild deer and bears in the forest coming down with cancer or diabetes; tigers and zebras in the jungle don't have high cholesterol or suffer heart attacks. But many household cats, dogs, and commercially raised livestock do. As far back as 1930, researchers at the Institute of Clinical Chemistry in Lausanne studied the immediate effects that eating cooked foods has on our bodies. They found that our bodies immediately respond to cooked food by increasing the number of white blood cells, a process known as "digestive leukocystosis." Generally, a jump in white blood cells is the body's normal response to viruses, infection, stresses, or other toxic invasions. Even foods that were not specifically cooked, yet are highly refined, such as white flour, sugar, or rice and other processed foods such as homogenized and pasteurized milk as well as any foods with added preservatives, created a noticeable increase in white blood cells. Keep in mind that highly processed foods were introduced into our culture in the 1930s, and that statistics show meteoric rises in cancer rates since that decade.

If our white blood cells are responding to the cooked and/or processed foods we eat, they are less available to us for when we really need them: to fight and eradicate disease. What these researchers also found, however, is that when we consume unprocessed, uncooked natural foods, this response does not occur. When we eat raw plant foods, we allow those resources to do their job and keep our immune systems strong.

> **The more you eat raw foods, the more your body starts to crave them, over anything else.** —MK

Essentially, when you eat cooked and processed foods, you lose nutritional benefits, sap your body's energy and enzymes, and gain instead harmful compounds such as free radicals, trans-fatty acids, and in the case of fried or grilled foods that are subjected to very high temperatures, carcinogens.

What About Meat?

In response to first hearing about the raw food diet, people often exclaim something like, "No problem . . . I *love* sushi!" Or they think beef tartare is on the menu. But consider for a moment our biological build—the structure of our intestines, the shape of our teeth—versus that of a tiger or a wolf. Not only do true carnivores have claws and fangs, but they also have very short intestines that allow them to eliminate the meat they eat very quickly. Humans have extremely long intestines; meat takes so long for us to digest that it often putrefies in our systems before we can expel the waste, thereby releasing toxins into our bloodstreams. As reported in the *New England Journal of Medicine* (323 (1990): p. 1664; *Cancer Research* 54 (1994): p. 2390), studies at Harvard and elsewhere on tens of thousands of women and men reveal that regular meat consumption increases the risk of colon cancer by as much as 300 percent. A health researcher at the Harvard School of Public Health recently commented that only two years on a high meat program such as the Atkins diet "could initiate a cancer. It could show up as a polyp in seven years and as colon cancer in ten" (*Nutrition Action Healthletter* January/February 2004). And what about heart disease? A study of 24,000 people, as reported in the *American Journal of Clinical Nutrition* (R. Phillips; 1978), found that the rates of heart disease for lacto-ovo vegetarians were one-third that of meat eaters; for vegans (vegetarians not eating eggs or dairy) the rate was one-tenth. There have been many studies since reporting similar trends.

If you do a little further research, you might learn, as we finally did, that meat consumption is not necessary or even remotely ideal for building a strong body. Read John Robbins's *Diet for a New America,* or his more recent book, *The Food Revolution,* where among all the other extraordinarily valuable information, he shows how vegetarians not only have much longer life expectancies, but fare far better in physical endurance and strength testing. He gives a long list of examples, including repeat Ironman Triathalon winners, world record-holding body builders, and Olympic gold medalists, such as Edwin Moses, who went eight years without losing a race. Yes, they're all vegetarians. For any skeptics, every claim he makes is well documented by legitimate research cited in the extensive footnotes. He also reveals the immense power behind the meat and dairy industries and the millions they spend on advertising and public relations in a truly eye-opening way.

> **In my perfect world, *Diet for a New America* would be a standard textbook in our schools, and *Fast Food Nation* would be like *The Catcher in the Rye*—no child would get past the eighth grade without reading it. People should eat whatever they want, but they should at least have a basic understanding of exactly *what it is* they are eating.** —SM

Despite whatever controversies may exist over any of these findings, doctors and scientists at least all pretty much agree that people should be adding *more* raw fruits and vegetables to their diets. Slowly this basic information is making its way out into the mainstream, allowing people to see that they have different options when it comes to diet and health.

Eating raw foods is not about sacrifice at all. It's about feeding your body the freshest, most natural and nourishing fuel. Your tastes will change as you go. If we're walking down the street on a cold and rainy day, maybe feeling bummed out about something and also a bit hungry—what do we crave? Green juice, salad, or maybe an avocado. Really! Those become the new ultimate comfort foods, because intellectually, emotionally, and instinctually we have learned that those are what *really feed* us and make us feel taken care of. That and a healthy dose of sunshine—nothing else makes you feel more alive!

If you fancy yourself a true meat lover, proudly call yourself a 'carnivore,' if your favorite way to eat roast chicken is to put the carved carcass on a plate and pick off all the meaty little bits with your fingers (this was mine!) or pick up a lamb chop with your fingers so you can gnaw off the bits closest to the bone (mine too!), then you should not think it impossible that you could very happily exist as a nonmeat eater, as I do now. People often say, 'I need meat to stay strong' or 'I couldn't live without the occasional burger.' Believe me, you can if you want to and it feels really good. Even the most purely grass fed, coddled beef from a cow that was sung to throughout its entire happy and hormone-free life, served on a freshly baked organic bun, can become unappealing very quickly. I can imagine, in an abstract way, that it would probably be very tasty, but my body really just doesn't want it.   —SM

Clear Eyes

Healthy skin, glossy hair, radiant eyes—yeah, we know, these are the characteristics that the American Kennel Club looks for in a championship dog. But it's also how raw foodists recognize one another (when not seated around the dinner table, that is).

Iridescent eyes, in particular, give it away. To some, they may be windows to the soul. But raw foodists believe that they are also peepholes to a person's state of health. Spots and irregularities in the eyes, according to the homeopathic study of iridology, are indicative of and correlative to various illnesses.

On the flip side, the more living enzymes you consume, the more you eradicate disease and cleanse your body. Your glowing eyes reflect this internal improvement, outer beauty increasing in ratio to inner beauty. On a raw diet, the color of your irises can even change, becoming lighter and exposing a broader stratosphere of hues.

A raw diet filled with antioxidants can also help improve vision and even prevent future diseases. For instance, if you have a family history of cataracts, eliminating cooked fats from your daily menu also rids the capillaries in your eyes of clogs.

Plagued by puffiness or dark circles under your eyes? Both can be improved with the right intake of potassium (for lid edema) and organic sodium (for those grim under-eye smiles). Just remember there's no magic pill, living or otherwise, for not getting enough sleep.

STOCKING UP/ INGREDIENTS

If you've been inspired to give raw foods a go, or even just slowly want to replace more processed and cooked foods with healthier options, this section can help get you started.

That motto of the Boy Scout brotherhood comes to mind: "Be Prepared." If you want to transition to eating raw foods, the more you can stock your cupboards with good stuff, the easier it will be. You can do it gradually, or you can have fun going through your cupboards and tossing out (or giving away) all the things you don't want anymore. Try it. It feels good! Those boxes of hardened brown sugar that you last baked with two years ago? The refined and processed oils, chemically preserved condiments, sugar-filled jams and jellies, artificial sweeteners? Toss 'em.

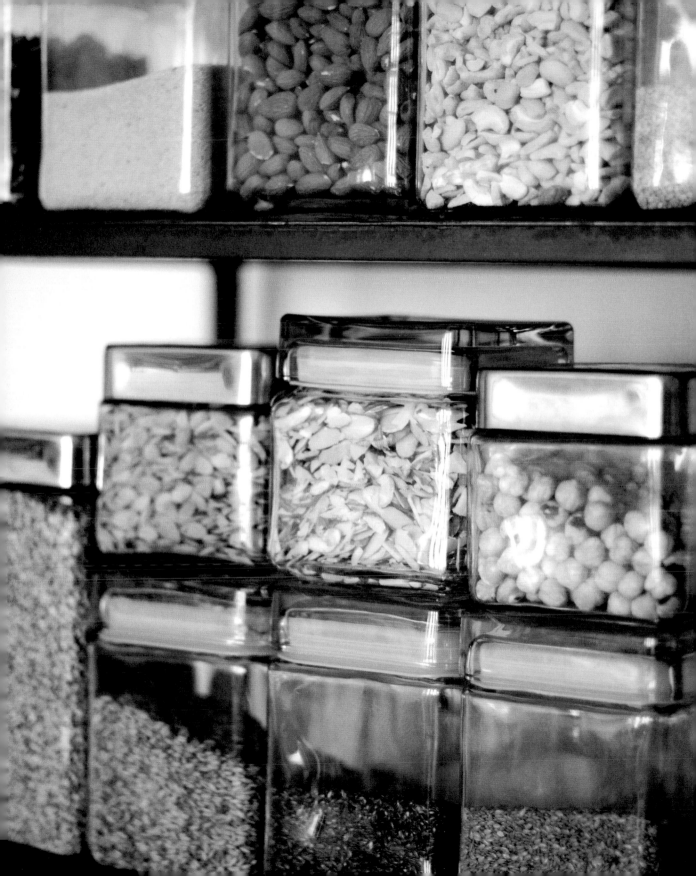

Below we've included a partial list of the things that you might want to start adding back into those clean cupboards, counters, and refrigerators. You'll find more discussion on many of these ingredients throughout the recipe chapters. For more detail on where to buy many of these items, check Sources on page 357.

Carob: Carob powder is ground from long pods that are grown in the Middle East. It has a sweet, caramel-like flavor and is very often used as a substitute for cocoa. It's high in minerals and B vitamins, with a small amount of protein and a smaller amount of fat. Carob is also an excellent source of pectin (which makes it a good colon cleanser, for those who are interested). Many carob powders are toasted, so look for one labeled "raw." You can find it at some health food stores or order online.

Cocoa powder and raw cacao: Cocoa powder is not raw (it has been roasted). But it still has a lot to offer (aside from amazing chocolate flavor!) and you can always substitute carob powder, or use a combination of both, if you are not comfortable with the "cooked" version. Organic cocoa powder can be found at health food stores. Raw cacao beans, however, are less readily available, but worth seeking out. Add cracked cacao pieces to Vanilla Ice Cream, page 253, for bittersweet chocolate chip ice cream, stir them into cookies or even shakes. See page 203 for more information on the benefits of cocoa and raw cacao.

Coconut butter: In comparison to other fats, the medium-chain fatty acids in coconut butter are more likely to be used for energy and less likely to be stored as fat. In addition, it has powerful antibacterial and antiviral properties and is particularly good for boosting immunity. We use a lot of coconut butter in our desserts, and love to add heaping tablespoons of it to many of our shakes (and rub it on our skin instead of lotion). Coconut butter's melting point is around 70°F, so it's more of a "butter" at cooler temperatures, and becomes an oil when the weather warms up. Just make sure it tastes and smells fresh before you add it to anything. See Sources, page 357, for more information on the best kinds to buy.

Coconuts: Many of our recipes call for young Thai coconuts. These are becoming more readily available in health food stores. You can also order them online, but the shipping is generally very expensive. The best source is your local Asian market. We also believe that pretty soon you will be able to readily buy fresh coconut water by the quart and fresh coconut meat by the pound, as more people discover the young coconut's amazing properties and taste. While it's not ideal, both the water and meat freeze very well. You can crack open coconuts in large batches when you have the time, and freeze the meat in zip-top bags and some of the water in quart containers for future use. We do this all the time at home. Just remember to leave room at the top of the container when freezing any liquids, as they expand.

Dried fruits: We like to keep dates, raisins, dried cranberries, and currants on hand for snacking. Adding pitted dates to shakes is a really great way to add sweetness and richness, and raisins, cranberries, and currants are all great in salads. It's easy to go overboard and eat a lot of dried fruits when you first start following the raw food lifestyle—we did—but they're not so easy to digest, so be careful. Also make sure the ones you buy are not treated with preservatives, like sulfur, or sweetened with refined sugars. When you're traveling or stuck at work for too long, however, having some dried papaya at your elbow is a far better option than any of the frightening offerings from most vending machines. Store dried fruits in glass jars or other air-tight containers in the cupboard or on the shelf. Dates, if you plan to keep them for longer than a week or so, stay fresh best in the fridge.

Fruits and vegetables: Of course, buy *organic*! Shopping at stores that carry only organic produce is best, but many markets carry both. It's always a good idea to check those little round stickers. There will be a 4- or 5-digit PLU number on it—when it's 5 digits and begins with the number 9, it's organic. Four digits means it's conventionally grown, and 5 digits beginning with the number 8 means it's been genetically modified.

That said, it's also very important to buy *locally*, especially from greenmarkets. And remember, many of them may not be *certified* organic, simply because the process for certification can unfortunately be costly and full of red tape (same goes for wines). But they still might be pesticide-free and sustainable. All you have to do is ask. Most vendors at farmer's markets aren't using genetically modified produce and/or spraying their crops.

If you're going to be eating your produce within a day or two, it's fine to keep it on the counter. For longer storage, most vegetables (and always greens and herbs) should be stored in the humidity-controlled bin in the fridge. Fruits are best left on the countertop or windowsill; it's especially helpful to keep organic citrus in the sunlight. Mushrooms should be wrapped in a paper bag in the refrigerator so they can breathe—they'll get slimy fast if stored in plastic. With avocados, it's generally a good idea to buy them unripe and let them ripen on your counter (or in a warm, inducing place, like a paper bag with an apple or banana, if you need to speed up the process). If you try to buy very ripe avocados, too often you'll find that they're all bruised and brown inside from being squeezed and bounced around by produce-fondling shoppers and careless stockers.

Keep in mind that freezing things is better than letting them go bad and throwing them out! When those pretty blushed apricots are in season, you might get a bit carried away and buy a whole bunch of them, only to find they are going too soft before you can eat them all. Pit and slice them and put them in a plastic freezer bag. While freezing causes some nutrient loss, it's minimal enough that we should make use of this handy, modern-day convenience. It also means that in the colder months, when those apricots are a distant memory, and you're getting a bit tired of apples and pears, you can thaw them out to eat plain or use in a shake (or cocktail!). They're also good to take on road trips or to the office, since they'll be perfectly thawed by the time your hunger pangs call.

Manna bread: Manna bread is an organic, muffin-like bread comprised of sprouted grains and baked at very low temperatures. The Nature's Path brand can be found in the freezer section of most health food stores. The cinnamon date variety is our favorite. It *may* not be 100 percent raw, as we're not sure of the exact temperatures to which they heat the bread, but it's a really great snack to have around, especially if you are transitioning, and it is leaps and bounds better than baked breads made of refined flours.

Miso: Miso is a fermented paste generally made from soybeans, barley, or rice and commonly used as a seasoning in China and Japan. While the ingredients aren't raw, the fermentation process makes it *live,* or full of natural digestive enzymes and other microorganisms that aid in digestion. It is also full of B vitamins and contains all eight of the essential amino acids that are needed to assimilate protein. Our favorite brand of miso is South River Miso, which you can find at many health food stores.

Nama shoyu: Nama shoyu is a particular kind of soy sauce that has not been pasteurized. It is made from cultured soybeans and wheat and aged for months (or even years). Without preservatives and full of enzymes, it has a great flavor and is the only soy sauce we use. You can find it at any health food store or online.

Nut and seed butters: Raw almond butter is a staple of ours, both as an ingredient and a snack. It's expensive, so if you find it on sale, buy a lot at once. We like to eat it on Manna bread (see previous page) with sea salt and raw honey, or on celery with raisins. Other nut butters, like cashew or macadamia, are also amazing, but usually even more expensive than almond butter. Making your own nut butters is possible but not practical—it's kind of messy and not as straightforward as it might seem.

Raw tahini (sesame seed paste) is also a great ingredient for making hummus, one of the easiest, fastest, and tastiest recipes for having on hand when the munchies strike (page 216). It's also good for creamy, herbal salad dressings.

Nutritional yeast: Grown specifically for its nutritional value (hence the name), nutritional yeast has a savory, almost cheesy flavor that is great to add to nut cheeses, crackers, and some sauces. It's very rich in vitamins, particularly B-complex vitamins, as well as essential amino acids. It can be purchased in bulk at many health food stores or online, and has a long shelf life (more than a year). Store it in an airtight container in the cupboard, and away from your pets. We left some in a bag on the counter once, and our cats tore it open and dragged it about. We came home to nutritional confetti all over the house.

Nuts and seeds: Space permitting, it's generally best to store your nuts and seeds in airtight containers in the refrigerator. Nuts can actually go rancid if exposed to too much light and they're left sitting around for too long. See page 43 for tips on soaking and dehydrating nuts, which makes them more digestible and familiarly crunchy—perfect for keeping in your office desk drawer or taking on trips. Almonds are our favorite snacking nut. Others good to keep around include Brazil nuts,

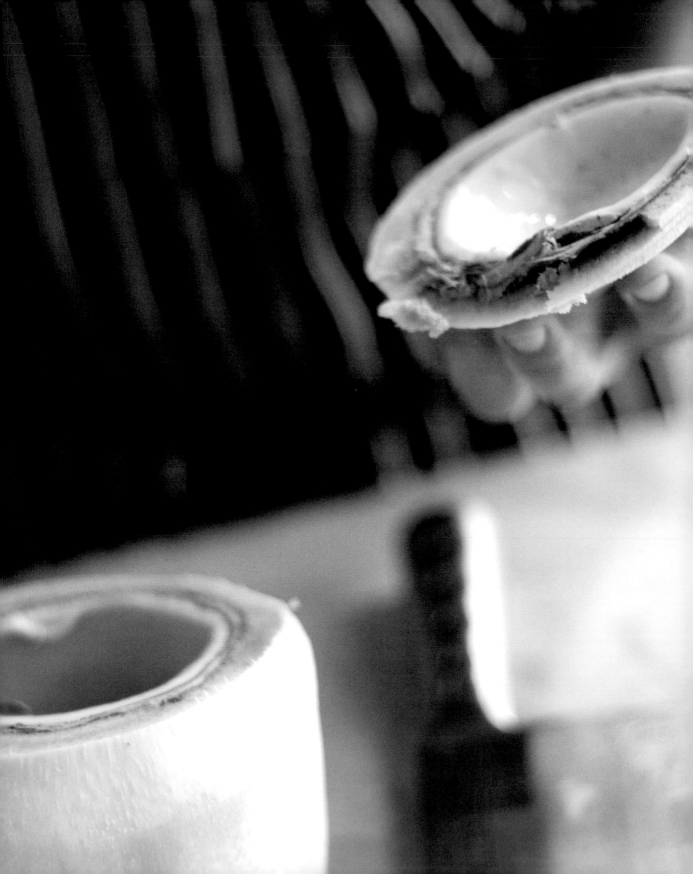

cashews, hazelnuts, pecans, pine nuts, pistachios, and walnuts. Make sure the nuts you are getting are fresh (as opposed to sitting around in a dusty bin opposite the yogurt-covered raisins). The busier the store, the better the odds that the nuts, as well as other ingredients, are fresh. Less popular nuts, as a rule, tend to be the most stale. Alternatively, online ordering is usually very reliable (see Sources, page 361).

As for seeds, we go through a lot of dark and golden flax, pumpkin, sunflower, and sesame seeds, and keep them on the shelves or in cupboards. While they look pretty in clear glass jars, it's always best to keep things away from light whenever possible. Hemp seeds, however, are best kept in the refrigerator. They are perfect on salads and sometimes we even just eat them plain with a spoon.

Olive and other oils: High-quality oils are not as easy to come by as one might think. As you might have guessed, we recommend only cold-pressed oils, but even some labeled as such may, in fact, be otherwise. Do your research. Either that or buy from small, artisanal producers or from raw food supply sources that generally have done the homework involved in investigating quality and purity concerns for you. A fairly good brand of olive oil is Bariani from California. It's cold-pressed and stone-crushed and they stamp each bottle with the harvest date and the bottling date. We are also partial to olive oils from Spain, having visited various producers and tasted some truly amazing oils on a recent trip there, and are seeking out cold-pressed, organically produced varieties to be imported and available in the United States. Among nut oils, macadamia is probably our favorite, with such a rich flavor that goes so well with so many different foods. Hazelnut, walnut, and Brazil nut oils can also provide an added dimension to many dishes. Be sure to store them in a cool, dark place, as olive and other oils can go rancid quickly.

Other oils we like to have around are generally more to be used as supplements, such as flaxseed oil and hemp seed oil. Both are very high in essential fatty acids, such as omega-3. These should always be kept in the refrigerator, and will (or should) always be sold refrigerated at the stores.

Salt: We love salt, but only the naturally harvested, sun-dried varieties, which are full of minerals and good things (see page 91 for more information). Fine sea salt is adequate for most recipes, particularly desserts, but if we had to buy only one texture, we would stick with the coarse version. Sprinkled on salads or finished dishes, the flavor from those crystals is amazing. We are also big fans of using salt in desserts—it draws juices and brings out other flavors rather intensely.

Sea vegetables: These may not sound like the most appealing thing when you're new to raw foods, but we think they taste amazing and they are extraordinarily good for you. We keep many varieties around to add to salads, particularly dulse, which has a nice smoky taste and does not need to be soaked first. You can just tear some up and add it to salads. Wakame, hijiki, and arame are also good varieties, and of course, nori for sushi rolls is undeniably tasty. In fact, nori is great for rolling up lots of ingredients as a snack: fill it with lettuce leaves, some Hummus (page 216) or Pignoli Ricotta (page 174), and sliced avocado and radishes. This is one of our favorite quickie lunches. Seaweeds are available at health food stores (look for untoasted nori). We buy Maine Coast Sea Vegetables and Emerald Cove brands most often, as they are the most readily available.

Spices, dried and fresh: It's always nice to have fresh flavoring agents around, such as chili peppers, lemongrass, ginger, and even galangal (similar to ginger, but a bit more exotic), if you can find it. Pureeing them into shakes and dressings, or juicing them, is easy and adds tons of character. Our favorite dried spices to have around are cumin seeds, cinnamon, star anise, coriander seeds, and dried chilies. You can buy all of these already ground, but it's better to purchase them whole and grind them per usage in a spice grinder.

Vanilla: An aromatic and very sexy flavoring, we use vanilla in most of our desserts and many of our shakes. Vanilla beans are costly and it's not especially easy to find organic ones, but the flavor the beans provide makes them worth the added expense (or minor deviation from all things organic, but you didn't hear that here). Vanilla extract is just that—the flavor extracted from the beans. You can find organic vanilla extract at any health food store, some specialty markets, or online (page 362).

Vinegars: The high acidity in many types of vinegar can actually destroy healthy bacteria in the intestines, so it's good to be moderate with its usage. Exceptions are raw apple cider vinegar, unfiltered brown rice vinegar, and umeboshi plum vinegar, all of which have more balanced acid levels. They're easily found at health food stores. We use other vinegars such as balsamic or mirin, the wine-based Japanese rice wine vinegar, in moderation, and only occasionally.

Natural Sweeteners

Agave nectar is derived, as the name indicates, from the agave cactus. Yes, that's the same plant that supplies tequila-makers with the raw ingredient. The nectar, a lightly textured, amber-hued liquid reminiscent in flavor of honey, isn't alcoholic, though. Agave nectar is extremely low on the glycemic index and is great for those who suffer from blood sugar disorders. Its mild flavor makes it a great ingredient in any shake or ice cream, and we use it to sweeten cocktails.

Dates, the oldest fruit, with the highest concentration of fruit sugars known to man, are quite simply a sweet temptation. Indeed some historians speculate that it was a date, not an apple, that provoked Adam's disobedience in Eden. After all, the fruit is origi-nally from the Middle East, the birthplace of both organized religion and cultivated crops. Today there are more than 400 varieties of dates, a highly prolific desert crop, though unfortunately we see only a few varieties in the United States and have more difficulty than we should buying them fresh. The big, juicy Medjool variety in particular seem an indulgence—they are sweet and decadent. If you have a Vita-Mix, they're effec-tive sweeteners for shakes and desserts when pureed thoroughly, though be sure to pit them first! You can also find date sugar (dehydrated and pulverized dates) at many health food stores. It works well in many dessert recipes or where we call for maple syrup powder.

Maple syrup has a caveat we want to mention at once: strictly, it's not raw. The sap that is gathered from the maple tree for a period of about three to four weeks in the spring is boiled to refine it, turning it into a thick syrup by steaming off excess water. We still like it, as long as it's 100 percent pure, and try to use it sparingly as it has a distinct flavor profile and is immediately recognizable if too much is used. Sweeteners usually play more of a supporting role than a leading one, so highlighting their distinct flavor may not be your goal. You can also buy maple syrup powder (simply dehydrated maple syrup) which we use in many dessert recipes (see Sources, page 360).

Raw honey, a collaborative product of flowers and bees, contains both fructose and glucose, is even sweeter than sugar, and is absorbed directly into the bloodstream. It is also rich in essential amino acids and nutrients, particularly amylase, which breaks down sugar and is heavy on the B-complex vitamins as well as C, D, and E. Be sure to use raw and unfiltered honey, however, which retains protein-rich bee pollen, over the heated and filtered brands. Honey that has never been heated will generally be solid at room temperature—if you can pour it, it's probably been heated, at least to some degree, and should really not be labeled "raw."

Stevia, a native South American herb that is cousin to the chrysanthemum, contains no sucrose. Instead, it has glycosides, which burst on the palate like an Olympic runner hits the track. The flavor of stevia is approximately 300 percent sweeter than conventional sugar, so the proverb "a little goes a long way" definitely applies here. It also has a slight anise overtone, making it more appropriate for some dishes than others. In addition, it's a good booster; we like to combine it with other sweeteners so that no one flavor dominates. Because it has no effect on blood sugar, stevia is a wonderful addition to the pantry of the raw foodist as well as anyone suffering from diabetes, yeast diseases like candidiasis, or gum disease. As with most herbs, stevia is easy to grow; we tend to our own in the small garden we have behind the outdoor seating at our restaurant. You can also find stevia in liquid or powdered form, but you'll only find it as a supplement. Unlike saccharine and aspartame, all-natural stevia—go figure—is not approved for commercial use as a sweetener, as it's not yet very widely distributed. We usually use the powdered form that comes in packets at the restaurant and in the recipes. It seems to have a slightly more mild taste than the liquid and is easier to measure consistently.

Yacon syrup, tasting not unlike molasses, is derived from its eponymous root, which grows only in the Andean region that begins in Venezuela and continues throughout Peru to northern Argentina. The brown-skinned yacon has a long, narrow, and knobby appearance and a white, crunchy, and juicy flesh. It is high in ogilofructose,

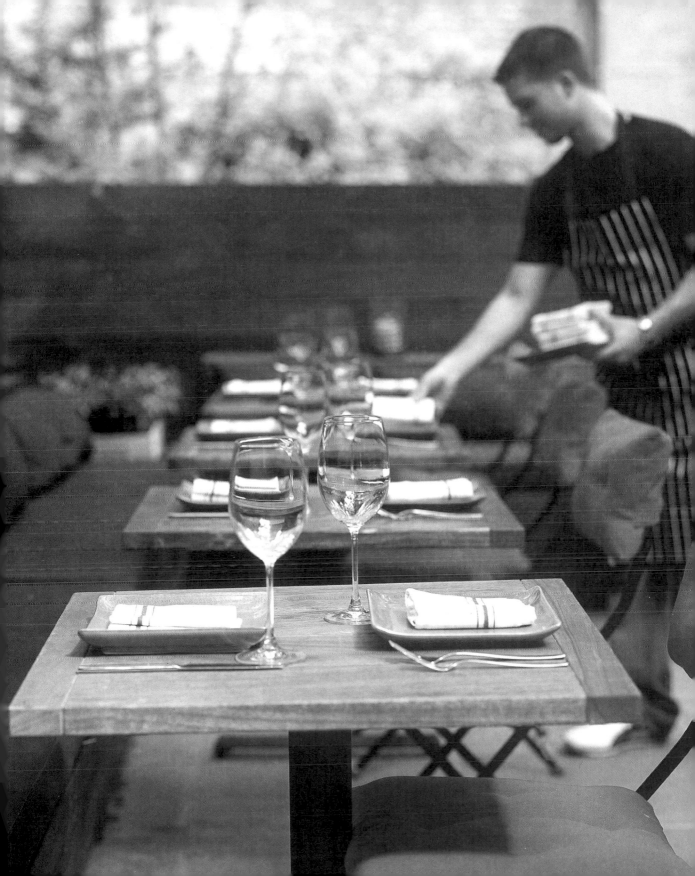

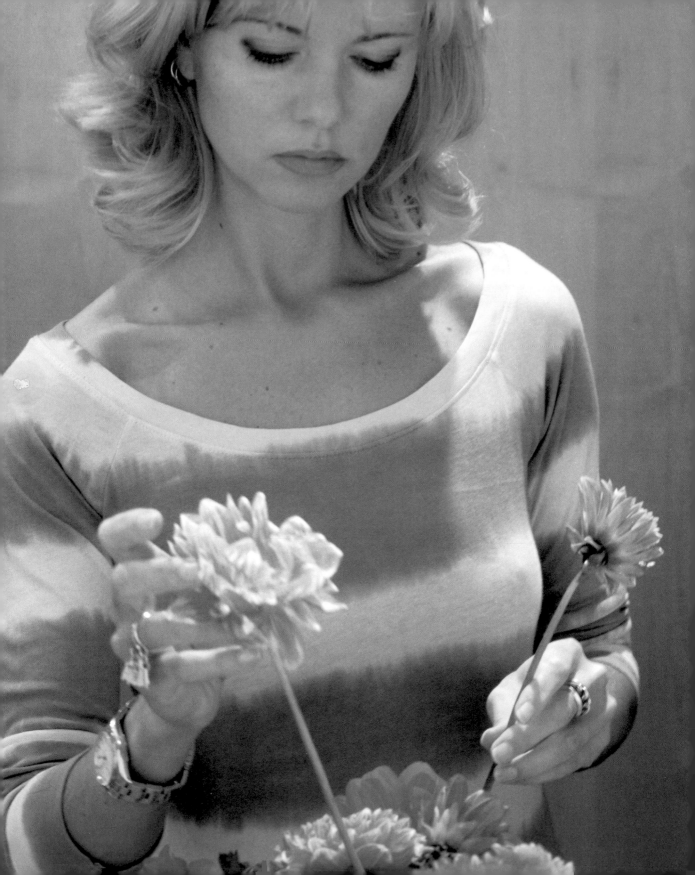

a natural sugar that intensifies when the root is dried in the sun. Peruvian farmers developed the syrup as an export product in order to boost rural incomes. Though far from well-known, the extracted yacon syrup, a jar of which has half the calories of an equivalent amount of honey, is inexpensive and appropriate for everybody from dieters to diabetics. As an added benefit, the ogilofructose characteristics also help the body to defend itself against osteoporosis and to retain beneficial bacteria in the colon. Since we came across this ingredient rather recently, it has not made it into our recipes, but you can easily substitute it for another sweetener in any recipe where a slightly molasses-like flavor would not be inappropriate, or add just a bit as a supplement. For example, you could add a tablespoon or two of yacon syrup in place of the same amount of maple syrup in a dessert or other recipe.

A Note on Supplements:

There are many supplements that get written about and recommended in raw food circles. We discuss many of them throughout these chapters and list sources in the back of the book, but there are still more to discuss—we'll just have to save them for another book. A few of our most recent favorites are goji berry juice, raw aloe vera juice, and PhytoNectars™. Be sure to fully research any supplements and herbs you use. Since they are unregulated (as they should remain), the onus remains with the consumer to evaluate what is or is not appropriate to take. As with foods, they also don't all have to be used all the time. One can easily get overwhelmed with all the research available and be tempted to stock up on all these pills, powders, and potions. But it's nice to try something for a while, see how you like it, and then move on to something else—particularly when the supplements are things that you can and really should be getting from natural food sources, such as straightforward vitamin and mineral supplements. The best supplements are the ones that are, in fact, *foods*—such as the high quality green powders and blue green algaes, or fruit concentrates, all made from food sources, not in a laboratory. In general, just keep an open mind, do a little careful experimenting, and pay attention to how your body feels.

Sweeteners: The Good, the Bad, and the Scary

First it was saccharine, said to cause cancer, that was taken off the market, then reinstated years later. Now aspartame, purported to be safe, is suddenly under suspicion as a "neuro-toxic food additive," according to the July/August 2004 edition of the *Well Being Journal*; three separate lawsuits have been filed in California against companies that produce and knowingly sell the allegedly dangerous sweetener in soft drinks to the consumer. Forget Big Tobacco—the next public health enemies just might be (and in our view, ought to be) Coke and Pepsi.

Consider this: If there's even a question about whether these substances are safe for you, why put them into your system? They might not turn out to be the culinary equivalent of Botox for your brain—though the experimental mice who keep falling off the treadmill and getting lost in the maze might squeak something different. As if being full of aspartame and other artificial sweeteners don't make diet soda bad enough, the acids in these sodas in particular leach vital minerals from your body, including calcium from your bones.

Of course, because we believe that the only things that should be processed are legal papers, we're not fans of commercially bleached, mineral-free white sugar either. According to *Eating for Beauty*, written by our friend and raw food expert extraordinaire, David Wolfe, "Heroin is produced by taking the juice of a certain type of poppy and refining it into opium, then morphine, and finally into heroin. Refined sugar is produced from taking the juice of sugar cane or beet and refining it into molasses, then brown sugar, and finally into white sugar." While Wolfe probably does not mean that sugar causes quite the same destruction (or high) as heroin, diets very high in refined sugar have been shown to have dramatic and behavior-altering effects on both children and adults, and it is not so far-fetched to think of it as a drug of sorts. Consider that the next time you see a child drinking one of those 20-ounce Cokes, containing 15 teaspoons of refined sugar—that's almost one-third of a cup!

The harvesting of sugar also destroys natural habitats (although some is sustainably raised and organically produced). Perhaps even worse, however, is corn syrup. Evil stuff. To get a good lesson on why, read the section entitled, "The Cornification of America and the World" in David Jubb and Annie Padden Jubb's excellent *LifeFood Recipe Book*. This was the very first book we read about raw and living foods, and it's what first got us hooked.

Fortunately, there are a variety of health-inducing, all-natural sweeteners that we use that are not poisonous to the body nor the environment.

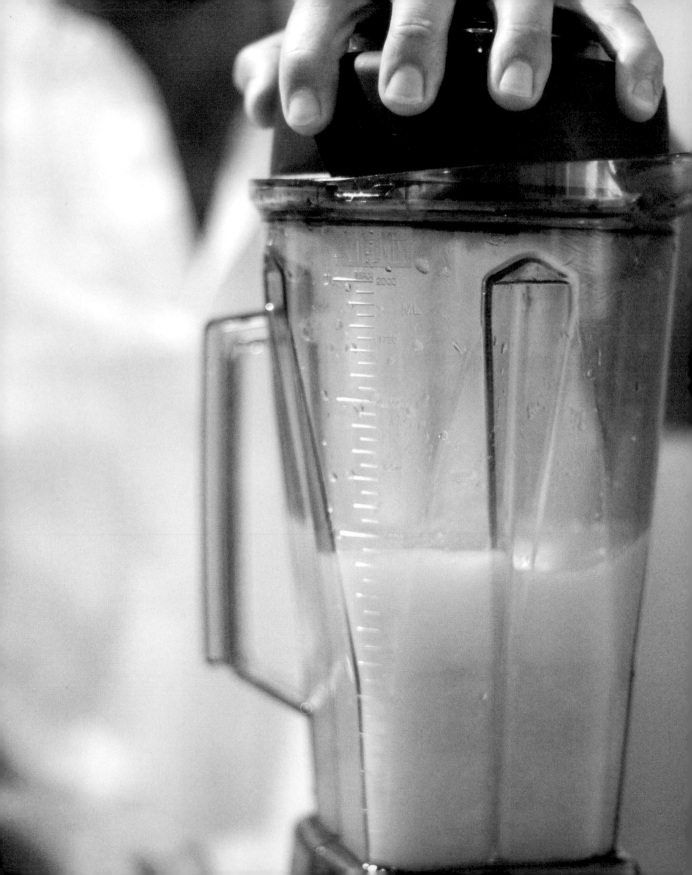

EQUIPMENT / TECHNIQUES

The equipment needed to prepare raw foods is minimal when you compare it with what you need to cook with heat. A few good tools, all reasonably priced, will allow you to make nearly every dish in this book, as well as create your own. Since any type of food preparation uses basic items like measuring cups and spoons, we have outlined only those special items that many kitchens may not have, but which are essential for the raw food lifestyle. These tools, along with a few basic techniques, form the basis for preparing most raw food dishes. Check Sources, page 357, for where to buy some of the more unusual items.

Equipment

Bamboo Sushi Mat These cost about $1.00. Well worth it!

Dehydrator Every raw foodist we know loves to experiment with dehydrating. For the first few months we had ours, it was always filled with some new recipe. In the cooler weather, it is also a great way to warm dishes slightly, or to thaw something from the freezer. Excalibur is, in our opinion, the best kind to get. The most practical model is the one with 9 shelves and 14-inch trays for $199. We have never seen another kind worth using. You will also need Teflex sheets, which have to be purchased separately. These are nonstick sheets to use when you are dehydrating something wet, like cracker batter. Otherwise, you can place foods like nuts directly on the mesh screens that come with the machine.

Food Processor Although it is possible to use the Vita-Mix for nearly everything, it often ends up blending things too much. For example, pestos, many nut cheeses, and condiments are far better slightly chunky. The food processor will allow the ingredients to be "processed" but still retain some texture. We use a Cuisinart, but any high-quality model should also work fine.

Good Knives A good knife is a sharp knife. Sharp knives are actually much safer, as they are less likely to slip. Once you are used to really sharp knives, working with anything dull is a drag. There are so many great products on the market now, but we prefer Global, as they are lightweight, virtually indestructible, and also happen to look very nice! It's critical to keep your knives properly stored (a knife block is necessary if you have good knives and wish to keep them safe and in working condition). In addition to a large chef's knife, a strong paring knife is essential. For cracking open young coconuts, we recommend a sharp-edged cleaver; an inexpensive but quality Japanese variety is best. You will also find a heavy-duty serrated knife quite useful. If you want to spend a bit more on knives, go for a good ceramic chef's knife—ceramic knives are non-reactive with foods. While they may break if you drop them on a hard surface or chip if you try to crack a coconut with one, they also don't need to be sharpened on a regular basis and are a pleasure to handle as long as you use them with care.

Japanese Mandoline The plastic version of the more costly, stainless steel professional model, this is actually easier to use, clean, and store, making it practical for a domestic kitchen. We use them for anything that needs to be uniformly sliced, especially when we're working with larger batches. Mandonlines are very inexpensive, extremely handy, and carried in most kitchenware stores.

Microplane Grater or Zester This is a great tool for preparing quick citrus zest or for grating very small items, even spices like nutmeg.

Mini Prep Cuisinart makes a $35.00 mini food processor that is perfect for chopping or pureeing very small amounts of product. It is also practical for chopping single items, like ginger. We always end up using it at home, since it is so easy to set up and clean, and works fast and efficiently.

Nut Milk Bag Nut milks are so good to have for shakes and smoothies, or even on their own, that we strongly recommend taking the time to find and stock a few of these bags, so that your milks can be smooth and creamy. We tried, early on, to replicate the effect with cheesecloth and strainers, which works fine, but is much messier. If you want that silky, smooth finish, it's well worth straining your milks. These bags don't cost much at all and as long as they are washed properly, they can be reused.

Peeler Ceramic peelers are the most efficient kind, though any peeler will do as long as you have at least one of these necessary tools.

Spice Grinder These are inexpensive and very handy to have for grinding spices or flaxseeds. A coffee grinder works just as well (as long as you aren't also using it on a regular basis for actually grinding coffee—they are not easy to clean and you would end up flavoring everything with coffee!). You can also do without this and use your Vita-Mix with the dry blade for grinding spices and nuts, but we find it's very convenient to have one of these handy for smaller batches.

Spiroli Slicer You don't have to get one, but they're very cool if you want to make squiggly noodles, and for only $25–$30, why not? A Japanese mandoline works fine for julienne or wide strips, but the spiral slicer makes nice curly fettuccini-like pieces from squash or zucchini.

Vita-Mix This is the turbo-charged version of the blender, making most domestic machines look like they are just for play. Ours gets daily use, often multiple times. Its power is essential and more than welcome when blending a thick shake, preparing Brazil nut milk, or even making your own nut butters. Its cost is higher than most blenders (about $400), but it will outlast any other type and will simplify your life and make your food preparation faster. It comes with an extremely thorough and useful manual, which we recommend you take the time to read to get the most from this essential tool.

Techniques, General Tips, and Guidelines

Coconuts For guidelines on cracking open coconuts, see page 64. Also keep in mind that you will often want to have on hand more coconuts than you think you might need for any particular recipe. Depending on the age of the coconut, some have very thick meat inside, while in others the meat is very thin and soft. While the latter is perfectly good for blending, you would not be able to cut noodles from these younger coconuts. That's another reason why it's a good idea to store extra fresh coconut pieces in the freezer. (See the note on coconuts in Stocking Up/Ingredients, page 25).

Dehydrating We provide guidelines in the book for the length of time various fruits, nuts, and crackers need to dehydrate. However, these times will *always* vary to some extent, depending on various factors such as the humidity in the air, as well as how many other items are in the dehydrator at the same time (the more wet stuff you have in it, generally the longer it takes). Dehydrating times will also vary depending on the exact thickness of the ingredients, so keep in mind that the times noted in the recipes are just guidelines. The best thing to do is to check frequently on the progress; over time, you'll get a feel for how long things take. The good news is, since many recipes do require a good bit of time, it's fairly difficult to *over*-dehydrate something.

Also keep in mind that when you season something *before* it goes in the dehydrator, it will come out much more strongly seasoned, as all the flavors will have been concentrated.

Dehydrating nuts Once nuts have been soaked, they may be more digestible, but are not really the most exciting thing to eat or add to a dish as is, all wet and soggy. For recipes that call for plain chopped nuts, we usually indicate "preferably soaked and dehydrated." If you don't have time, raw nuts are okay. Otherwise, it's nice to have already soaked and dehydrated nuts on hand, particularly almonds and cashews. While it takes time, it takes very little effort to soak a bunch of almonds overnight and then drain them and spread them on a dehydrator tray—for almonds, leave them in at 115°F for 24 to 36 hours, until they are very dry and crunchy. Then let them cool down, and put them in an airtight container or zip-top bag and store in the refrigerator. They will keep for months this way, and are great for snacks and salads. Same for cashews. They also make a nice nibble (particularly with a glass of wine or a cocktail) if you toss them in a bowl with enough nut oil just to coat them and add a generous pinch of fine sea salt.

Serving temperatures When you prepare dishes ahead, make sure you allow the components enough time to come to room temperature (unless you want to serve them chilled, of course). Coldness mellows the flavors. For example, when making the Red Beet Ravioli, you can make the filling and sauces ahead, but the dish will not taste as good if the cheese is *cold* and stiff when you assemble and serve it. If you haven't allowed enough time for something to come to room temperature on its own, you can generally warm it by putting it in the dehydrator, or also by immersing the container (sealed) in a bowl of lukewarm water.

Soaking nuts Soaking nuts in filtered water, then draining them and rinsing them again, makes them more digestible and removes bitter flavors without requiring the nuts to be roasted. The soak-drain-rinse cycle also takes away the enzyme-inhibitors that exist in the skin. These enzyme inhibitors are actually what allow nuts (and seeds and legumes, for that matter) to stay dormant until they are soaked, and ready to sprout and grow. It is nature's way of preserving their life force so they can reproduce in the future.

For the most part, we'll give you soaking times in the recipes, but it's basically a simple formula—the denser (harder) the nut, such as almonds, hazelnuts, and pistachios, the longer you need to soak them (4 to 8 hours). Medium-soak nuts such as Brazil nuts, pecans, and walnuts have more oils and become saturated more easily

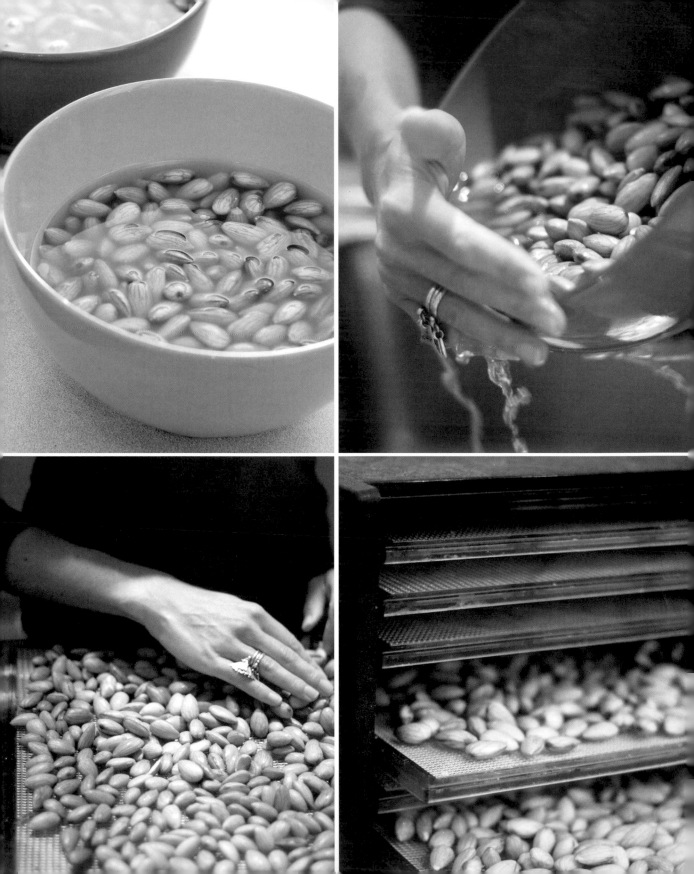

(2 to 4 hours). Short-soak nuts such as cashews, macadamias, and pine nuts, don't have those problematic inner skins and so require less time; soaking these too much can reduce their natural, life-affirming oils (1 to 2 hours is all you need). However, it's fine to soak any of these overnight if that is convenient. Just keep in mind that the longer they soak, the more waterlogged they become and you may need to use a bit less added water than called for in the recipe. Also, when you soak nuts, often one or two (or more) will rise to the top—it's a good idea to discard these floaters as it usually means they have gone rancid.

Sweetener substitutions If we call for a particular sweetener in a recipe that you don't have on hand or prefer not to use, you can generally substitute something else. Some raw foodists prefer not to use maple syrup, as it's technically not raw. For most of our recipes that call for maple, an ideal substitute would be a mix of agave nectar and another sweetener such as yacon syrup or dates, both of which would add a bit of the rich, caramel flavor that maple provides. Agave on its own will usually work fine, but keep in mind that it's a very neutral flavor. You can also add more stevia to recipes, if you want to keep your calories or sugar intake lower.

Water in recipes Many of our recipes call for water to be added to a mixture in the blender or food processor. We generally mention a range and indicate that you may need more or less. The amount will vary for a few reasons. One is that when we call for soaked nuts, they may absorb more or less water depending on the exact amount of time they were soaked, and so will require more or less *added* water to reach a certain consistency. Also, with these recipes, precise measurements are generally not required, and we call for things like nuts and other ingredients in cup measurements. Dry ingredients are more precise when measured by weight, but it's not that convenient to pull out a scale and weigh everything. A cup of whole macadamia nuts will have less in volume than if you are measuring macadamia pieces, so for this reason too, ingredients like added water or the amount of salt or other seasonings may vary a bit. These recipes are not set in stone, so if something doesn't feel or taste right, adjust it as you see fit or according to your own taste preferences.

Our recipes specify "filtered" water, but distilled water (which is cheaper than other bottled varieties) is fine too, if you don't have a home filtration system. If you do use tap water, just be aware that it's your body that will be doing the filtering!

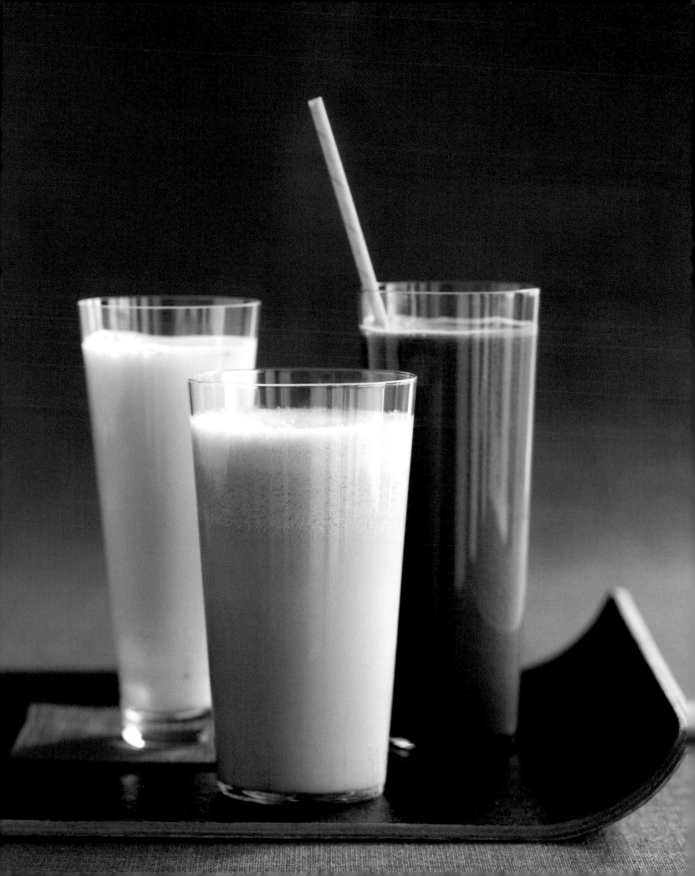

NUT MILKS AND SHAKES

Someday soon, you will likely be able to buy fresh or frozen nut milk at your local organic market; actually, you already can at our take-out in New York, and in certain stores in California. However, until they become as universal as tofu, there's always the homemade route.

Nut Milks

Nut milks are exactly what they imply—dairy-free, liquid refreshment gleaned from ground nuts. They're very easy to make, once you get the hang of it, and totally nutritious, with no hormones or antibiotics! In addition to common and familiar nuts such as macadamia, cashew, pecan, and almond, you can also use sunflower seeds, pepitas (pumpkin seeds), sesame seeds, and hemp seeds to make milks. A Vita-Mix, or other high-powered, high-speed blender is strongly recommended—conventional blenders just won't do the trick, as they generally don't have the power to really pulverize the nuts.

Some nut milks, such as almond or Brazil nut, require straining. When you do this, you can use multiple layers of cheesecloth, or you can look for a nut milk bag, which is, as you might guess, a fine-mesh bag made specially for straining nut milks (you can find them online; see Sources, page 357). When you strain the milk, squeeze the liquid out of the bag or cheesecloth into a glass bowl or other container. The pulp that remains can actually be used as an ingredient: you can dehydrate it and use it as a flour to make crusts for desserts (see chapter 5) or crackers (see chapter 7). Other, creamier nuts, such as macadamias or pecans, blend right into a smooth milk, and are a bit easier to handle.

When making nut milks, you might have to run the blender for a long time, which warms it up. If you're not planning to chill the liquid in the refrigerator before serving, simply use a bit less water and then, after it's thoroughly pureed, blend in some ice cubes to cool it down. You also don't always have to soak the nuts for as long as we recommend, but generally the longer they are soaked the more easily and quickly they will liquefy.

In general, nut milks will keep 2 days (or a bit longer if kept very cold) in a covered container in the refrigerator. The milk may separate, especially if you've added coconut butter, in which case just give it a good shaking or a quick whirl in the blender before serving.

If you find yourself with a lot of extra nut milk on hand, pour it into ice cube trays and freeze it. Transfer the frozen nut milk cubes to a zip-top bag and return to the freezer. You can use them to add richness to fruit shakes or extra frosty creaminess to already creamy shakes.

Shakes

As opposed to nut milks, you can usually make great shakes with any standard blender. Just be careful if you're using certain ingredients. For instance, we wouldn't recommend putting dried figs in a regular blender, since they could get caught in the blades and damage the motor.

Fruit shakes are easy and filling, and you can make them with just about anything. All you need to start is a liquid base—coconut water, fresh citrus juice, a juicy fruit such as watermelon, or nut milks—for a creamy shake. Oranges are great because you don't have to squeeze them. Just cut away the peel and dump them in, seeds and all. The seeds from organically grown citrus are good for you, as is the fiber from the pulp and any of the white pith you leave on.

There are endless variations; we have provided recipes for some of our favorites, which you can use as a guideline for creating your own. You can blend almost any fruits with nut milks to make a creamy snack. Try white or yellow freestone peaches, or mixed berries. You can also make a refreshing cooler by blending kiwis, strawberries, raspberries, coconut water, and a touch of lime; or blend fresh orange juice with almond milk for a drink that tastes almost eerily like those orange creamsicles from an ice cream truck. Note: When using raspberries and blackberries, run the blender a bit longer to break up the seeds. They're good for you, but not much fun when they get stuck in your teeth. For chillier shakes, add a few ice cubes (ideally made with filtered water), or buy extra fruit to cut up and keep in the freezer. We like to buy lots of bananas at once, wait until they are really ripe (and sweet) with little brown spots, then peel them, cut them in chunks, and store them in zip-top bags in the freezer. Using frozen banana instead of fresh gives smoothies more of an ice-cream shake quality.

Most of our shake recipes specify a natural sweetener, usually agave nectar or stevia. The quantity depends on personal taste. As you know, fruits vary in sweetness, so it's a good idea to taste your shakes *as* you add sweeteners. For example, pineapples can be ultra-high in sugar content, in which case you may need less sweetener (or none), or they can be acidic and tart, in which case you might want to add more. Sometimes we use fresh, pitted dates to sweeten fruit shakes, or raw honey—these are good options if you don't like stevia (some people find the herb to have a slightly bitter or licorice-type taste). Choose your sweetener according to what you prefer or what you have on hand. In these recipes, you can substitute as you wish, keeping in mind, however, that you might not want to use brown dates or maple syrup in your pure white coconut shake if you care about the color. Agave nectar goes very well with tropical fruits, whereas raw honey and dates might be better suited to stone fruits, apples, pears, or berries.

We encourage adding a pinch of sea salt to everything, both sweet and savory. When you use the right kind, salt brings out flavors nicely and is good for you, too. We almost always add a bit of pure vanilla extract to shakes as well, just because we like the additional element of flavor it provides.

Shakes as well as juices are a great vehicle for many food supplements, such as tocotrienols, Peruvian maca, bee pollen, hemp protein, green superfood, blue green algae, and others. Keep in mind that not all supplements will match, flavor-wise, with your shake or juice, so it's a good idea to experiment a little with your combinations. We've provided information on supplements throughout this chapter and the juices chapter, but just check the index for the specific page if you can't easily find it. There are plenty of other supplements out there that we may not have mentioned—just be sure to do your research and see what works for you.

Most of these recipes make around 32 ounces, so in general they yield two 16-ounce servings or four 8-ounce servings.

Finally, remember that shakes are fun. Forget measuring and just taste as you go. You will get in the mix and never need to look at a recipe again.

Vanilla Brazil Nut Milk

SERVES 2 TO 4

Brazil nuts are one of the best sources of selenium, a mineral that is otherwise hard to come by naturally. Selenium is like the rebar on a high rise—it's the reinforcement for one of the body's most powerful antioxidants. The coconut butter isn't essential, but it's a healthy addition that provides flavor and richness. The lecithin gives the milk extra smoothness.

> "This milk is sweet, natural, and really good for you. —MK"

1 cup raw Brazil nuts, soaked 2 hours or more

4 cups filtered water

$1/4$ cup agave nectar or raw honey

2 tablespoons coconut butter

1 tablespoon vanilla extract

1 tablespoon lecithin (optional)

2 packets stevia

Pinch of sea salt

In a Vita-Mix or high-speed blender, blend the nuts and water on high speed for about 2 minutes, to make sure the nuts are thoroughly blended. Strain the milk through a nut milk bag or multiple layers of cheesecloth twice for smoothness. Rinse the blender cup and place the milk back in it with the remaining ingredients. Blend to combine thoroughly and taste for sweetness.

Variations

FOR CHOCOLATE MILK, add 3 heaping tablespoons of organic cocoa powder or carob powder, plus an additional packet of stevia or tablespoon of agave, to the blender along with the strained milk and other ingredients.

FOR STRAWBERRY MILK, add about 1 pint of washed and stemmed strawberries, plus an additional packet of stevia or tablespoon of agave, to the blender along with the strained milk and the other ingredients above.

Lecithin

A fatty substance that is naturally produced by humans, other animals, and plants, lecithin is actually a widely used commercial additive. Check the back of a tub of margarine or ice cream carton—it's probably in the ingredients. As a supplement made from soybeans, lecithin is a fat emulsifier, making things creamy, and it is a big help for vegans who like the texture of dairy foods but not the dairy itself. Lecithin also contains choline, a B vitamin that is mandatory in every infant formula on the market—it's that necessary for you. Lecithin and choline protect against memory loss and impairment, as they are components in brain cells and help manufacture neurotransmitters, and are so good for the liver that alcoholics are treated with high doses of the supplement. Be sure, however, to buy lecithin made only from non-GMO soybeans (that's soybeans that are not of the genetically modified Frankensoy variety—unfortunately soybeans are among the most widely tampered-with crops). It's sold as a powder (see Sources, page 359).

Water

We've heard it so many times we tend to ignore it. Our bodies are roughly three-quarters water, and it's pretty hard to regenerate cells, inside and out, if we're not getting enough liquid. At the restaurant, we use the Tensui purification system, which filters the water in the entire place—even the H_2O in the toilets is purified, though we don't recommend you drink it (even if you're a dog). The Tensui system is big in Japan and many hospitals use it. At home we don't have a water filtration system yet, though we plan on getting one. We drink Trinity water (the preferred raw foodie brand) or buy distilled water by the gallon for soaking nuts and seeds. The ideal source for your body, however, is fruits and vegetables. Cucumbers, celery, watermelon, tomatoes, and other juicy fruits and vegetables contain the purest water you can find! So if you're eating plenty of raw fruits and vegetables, theoretically you may not need the daily eight glasses of water recommended—that's for all the people out there that like to cook all the water out of their food, so they need at *least* that much to make up for it.

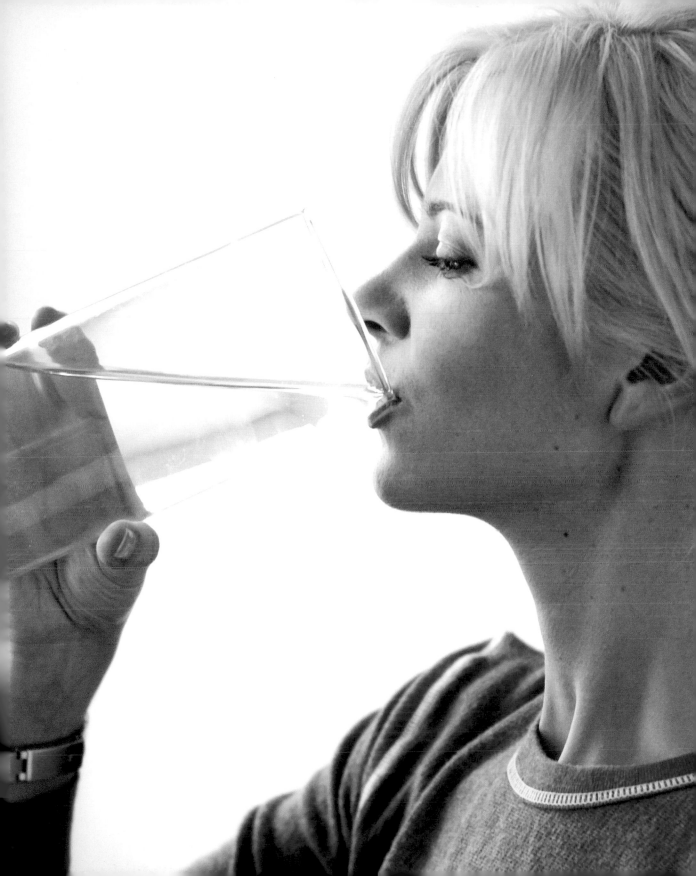

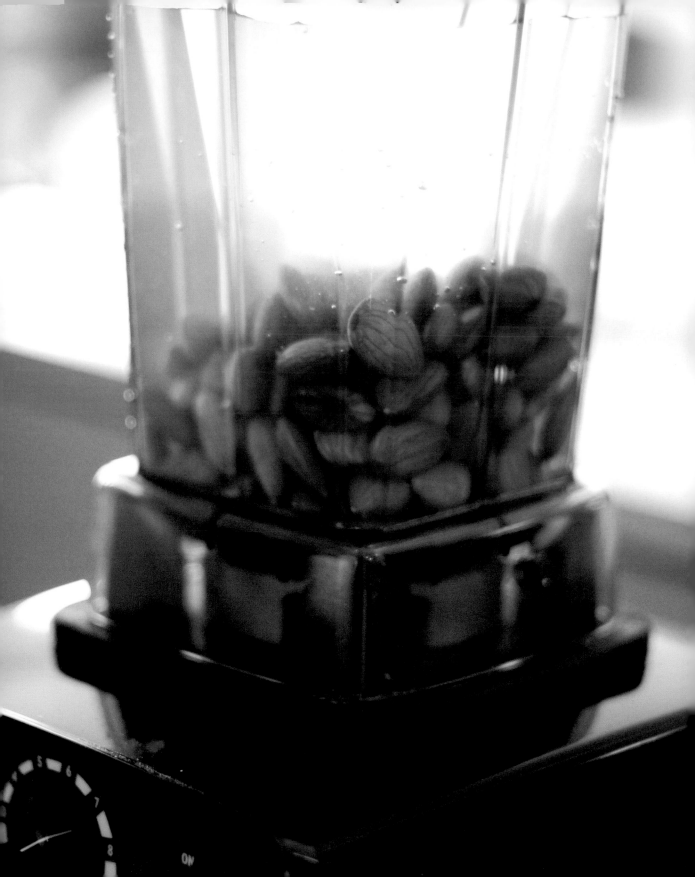

Almond Milk

Almonds are one of the only alkaline nuts, and an excellent source of vitamin E. At almost 20 percent protein, almonds are a satisfying snack, and *this* milk really *does* do your body good.

> " I love almond milk poured over both the maple cinnamon and cocoa versions of our buckwheat cereal (page 272). Before going raw, we used to drink a lot of soy milk—but do enough research on soy and you'll likely shift away from it too. " —SM

1 cup raw almonds, soaked 4 hours or more
4 cups filtered water
$^1/_4$ cup agave nectar or raw honey
1 tablespoon lecithin (optional)
Pinch of sea salt
A few drops of natural almond extract (optional)

In a Vita-Mix or high-speed blender, blend the nuts and water on high speed for about 2 minutes, to make sure the nuts are thoroughly blended. Strain the milk through a nut milk bag or multiple layers of cheesecloth twice for smoothness. Rinse the blender cup and place the milk back in it with the remaining ingredients. Blend to combine thoroughly and taste for sweetness.

30-Second Nut Milk

Here's how to make nut milk in a pinch, when you don't have time for (or just don't feel like) soaking and straining. You can use this as a substitute for regular nut milk in the shakes, or drink it straight up.

> "This is a very convenient alternative to making traditional nut milks and couldn't be easier. If you're trying to put on weight, as I was for awhile, add an extra tablespoon of nut butter for a richer milk." —MK

2 heaping tablespoons raw almond or cashew butter, or any other raw nut butter
2 cups filtered water
Pinch of sea salt
2 tablespoons agave nectar or 1 packet stevia
$1/2$ teaspoon vanilla extract
1 tablespoon coconut butter (optional)

In a blender, puree all ingredients until smooth.

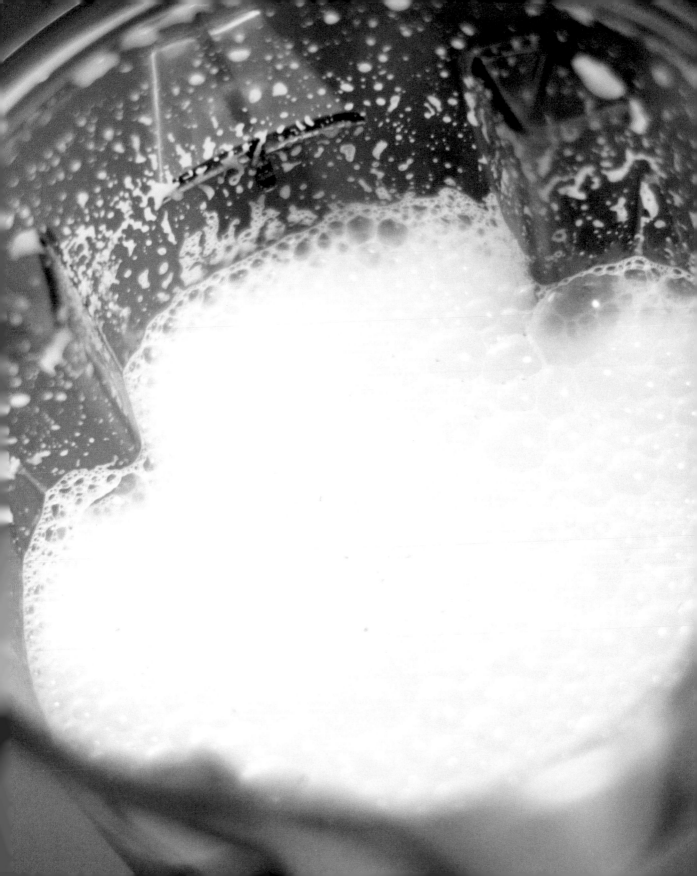

Dear Dairy

What you have suspected so long is true—we have given you the brush-off.

It's not that we don't love you. But we know what you do to us. You line our intestines with mucus, making it difficult for us to digest, assimilate, and eliminate our foods. You clog our arteries and give us respiratory and heart problems. You make us fat and congested and misplace our trust with slogans such as "Milk—it does a body good." Who really needs your trademarked mustache?

Not the majority of Asians, African Americans, and Eastern European Jews, who are lactose-intolerant. In short, an estimated 60 percent of society can't tolerate you intestinally, lacking the enzyme to digest your milk sugar. The rest of us get sluggish and fatigued when we consume you. From this standpoint, it makes sense since humans were not designed to process dairy products in the first place, particularly *pasteurized* dairy. After all, centuries ago we had our mothers to nourish us, and those who couldn't for some medical or biological reason relied on Dr. Nestle (he of the chocolate family who invented, believe it or not, infant formula).

We also don't like what's in you—low doses of antibiotics, steroids, and hormones that are supposed to keep you free from diseases and help you lactate longer, but in fact may cause *us* illness and resistance to beneficial bacteria in the long run. And then there's what's *not* in you. All those vitamins and calcium you're supposed to have? Green leafy vegetables like broccoli, kale, spinach have so much more. And convincing us that you're the key to avoiding osteoporosis? The nations with the highest intake of dairy, the United States, Sweden, and Finland, also have shown the highest rates of the bone degenerating disease. Why? Because it's the acidic conditions you create in us that makes our bodies pull the alkaline calcium *out* of our bones to neutralize the acid, leaving us with a net calcium defecit. Just check out www.milksucks.com for more information.

So we are giving you, and the myth that we need you, up. It's not without qualms— we might love the taste of ice cream, yogurt, and cheese like children. You and your byproducts just don't love us back, and that's the bottom line.

Cinnamon Maple Pecan Milk

SERVES 2 TO 4

If you don't want to use maple syrup, which isn't strictly raw, use agave nectar. This milk is yummy with the Maple Cinnamon Buckwheat Crispies cereal (page 272) if you're really a big fan of cinnamon. As with many nuts, it's best to keep shelled pecans in the refrigerator for longer storage.

> "This milk is nice in the fall and winter, as it always tastes somewhat festive to me—maybe because it reminds me of eggnog." —SM

1 cup raw pecans, soaked for 2 hours or more
3¹/₂ cups filtered water
¹/₄ cup maple syrup
2 tablespoons coconut butter (optional)
2 teaspoons vanilla extract
1 tablespoon lecithin (optional)
2 packets stevia, or an additional 2 tablespoons of maple syrup
³/₄ teaspoon ground cinnamon
Pinch of freshly grated nutmeg
Pinch of sea salt

In a Vita-Mix or high-speed blender, blend the nuts and water on high speed for about 2 minutes. Add the remaining ingredients and blend to combine. Taste for sweetness.

Creamy Macadamia Milk

SERVES 2 TO 4

Macadamia nuts are second only to Brazil nuts in selenium and very high in zinc, both important minerals. Macadamias are the richest source of the monounsaturated fat oleic acid, otherwise known as omega-9, beneficial for lowering cholesterol and protecting against heart disease. Like the fatty acids in coconut, those in macadamias help the body more efficiently metabolize fats and so, counterintuitively, are thought to promote weight loss.

> **I like this milk a bit richer, so I use 3 cups of water instead of the 4 that we usually use per cup of nuts—it's great to mix with fruits for creamy drinks. You don't really need to strain it, but we often do for a smoother liquid.** —MK

1 cup raw macadamia nuts, soaked 1 hour or more
3 cups filtered water
3 tablespoons agave nectar
2 tablespoons coconut butter (optional)
2 teaspoons vanilla extract
1 tablespoon lecithin (optional)
1 packet stevia
Pinch of sea salt

In a Vita-Mix or high-speed blender, blend the nuts and the water on high speed for about 2 minutes. Add the remaining ingredients and blend to combine. Taste for sweetness. Strain, if desired.

Pineapple Star Anise Lassi

SERVES 2 TO 4

Lassi is a traditional Indian shake made with yogurt. When you order one in a restaurant, the waiter will usually ask if you want it savory or sweet (the latter can also be made with mango). Our version is on the rich, sweet side.

> " Star anise is one of my favorite spices . . . like cinnamon but more exotic. You can make this with mango instead of pineapple—try adding a tiny pinch of ground cardamom instead of the star anise. " —MK

3 cups diced pineapple
1 cup macadamia milk
³/₄ teaspoon ground star anise

In a blender, puree all ingredients until smooth.

Sometimes You Feel Like a Coconut

The coconut has gotten a bad rap over the years. Coconut milk, flesh, and oil—all of which are actually good for you—at one time or another have been implicated in everything from an increase in heart disease to the melting of the polar ice cap.

All right, so the coconut really isn't being blamed for global warming, but there have been a number of unflattering reports in years past bad-mouthing a substance we would never recommend either: *hydrogenated* coconut oil. Yes, that kind is full of those evil trans-fatty acids. Remember the movie theater popcorn scare? While hydrogenated oils of *any* kind are truly destructive, the pure and unmolested coconut, from which we can cold-press the most amazing oil, could not quite recover from this PR nightmare. That is, until now. Coconut is in fact making a splashy comeback into mainstream media as a hot new "diet" food, with coverage in outlets such as *Vogue* magazine and trendy diet books.

The fact of the matter is that these undeservedly maligned fruits of the coconut palm, particularly the water that is cradled in fresh young coconuts, are incredibly healthy. Coconut water is low in calories, carbs, and sugars and is almost completely fat-free. Conversely, it's high in ascorbic acid, B vitamins, proteins, and electrolytes—nature's answer to Gatorade.

Fans of coconut water rave about the beautifying powers that range from restoring chapped lips to combating the appearance of freckles, sunspots, and skin cancers. Internally, the isotonic drink not only restores the body's electrolytic balance, it aids in the function of the gall bladder, kidney, liver, and thyroid. Keep in mind that the water from *young* coconuts is preferred. As the coconut matures, the amount of ascorbic acid is reduced and the sugars begin to concentrate and increase. At the restaurant and at home, we use young Thai coconuts. What you also see in the

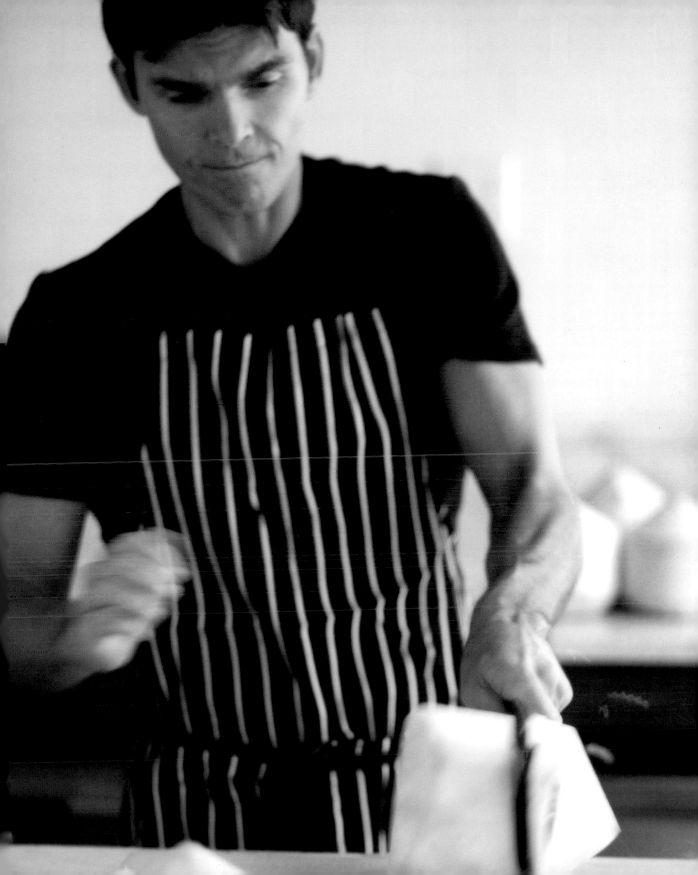

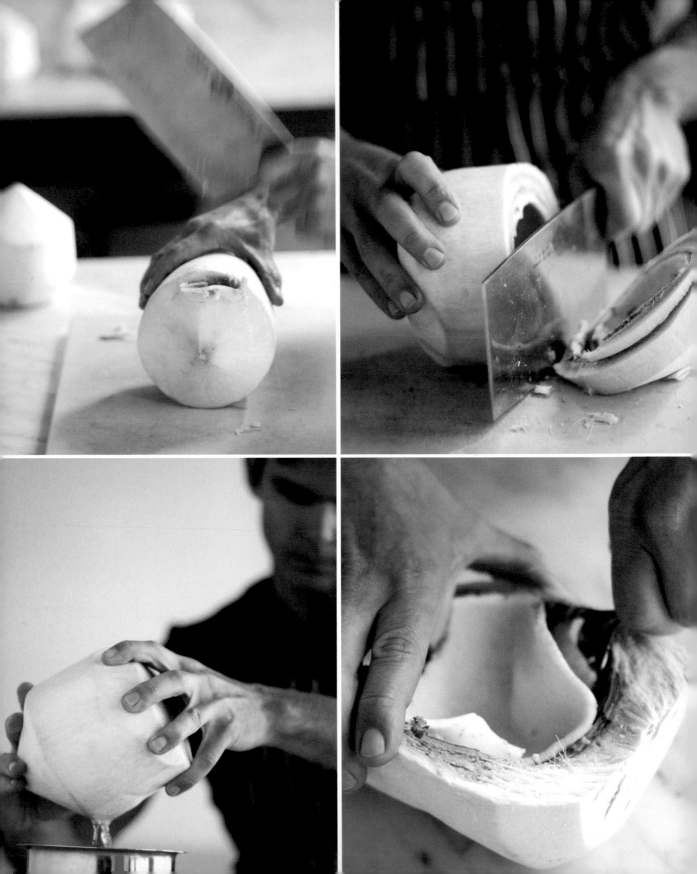

markets labeled as "coconut milk" is the extract of the grated flesh of the mature coconut, which generally comes pasteurized in a can, so it's not an ingredient we would use.

The whole young coconuts generally come with the husks trimmed down, so they sit flat with a pointed top. To open these coconuts, a cleaver is your best bet. You can use a chef's knife, but if you do, make sure it's an old, inexpensive one! Lay the coconut on its side, securing it so that it won't roll. Try not to hold the fruit with your free hand while you make the first cut (in case you have particularly bad aim!). Holding the knife high, bring it down sharply near the top of the coconut. The knife should sink in about one-third of the way, breaking through the inner shell. Quickly set the coconut upright so as not to lose the water to the cutting board. If you didn't succeed in breaking the inner shell, rotate the shell and try the technique again. Drain the coconut of its water into a blender or bowl, then use the cleaver or knife to finish cutting off the top to get at the meat.

The meat will range from very thin and very soft (sometimes even with a pale purplish hue in very young coconuts), to thicker and firmer. The firmer meat is best for recipes that call for noodles or pasta squares. Sometimes you have to open a few before you get one with nice firm meat, but the soft meat is perfectly good for sauces and smoothies, and coconut meat freezes beautifully, so all of it is good to use. The best way to get the firmer meat out is by using the back of a spoon to pry it from the sides of the coconut, then trim away any of the shell residue with a paring knife. Lay the pieces of coconut flat on a cutting board and slice into $\frac{1}{6}$-inch strips for dishes that call for coconut noodles.

We also like to use young coconut oil, or "butter" (see Sources, page 358). It's very important to buy only cold-pressed *virgin* oil, which is mechanically extracted from the young coconut meat. Only fresh, young coconut butter will have a smooth, coconutty or neutral flavor. Beware of any coconut butter that has a toasted sort of flavor—it's either made from dried or mature coconut or has gone rancid. While coconut butter is extremely stable, it's important to keep it in an opaque container away from heat and light. Its melting point is somewhere around 75°F, so don't be surprised in the warmer weather if you open a jar of coconut butter to find a liquid. At lower temperatures, it's more like butter (hence the package name of butter or oil). You can keep it in the refrigerator for longer storage, but then it's difficult to scoop it out neatly as it gets very hard.

The fat in coconut oil is made up of medium chain fatty acids, and as such is more likely than other fats to be used as an energy source rather than stored as fat. Many studies indicate that it boosts metabolism of fat and therefore aids in weight loss. Delicious as a flavor element, coconut oil/butter has other qualities and uses: it's terrific for removing eye makeup, or for moisturizing the skin.

> **Our cats are complete fools for coconut butter. I discovered this when they started licking my shins after I put it on as lotion, and also loitering around the bathtub like vultures waiting for me to use it to shave my legs. Now we feed them a little bit directly every day and they eagerly lick it up. And they still won't leave me alone in the tub.** —SM

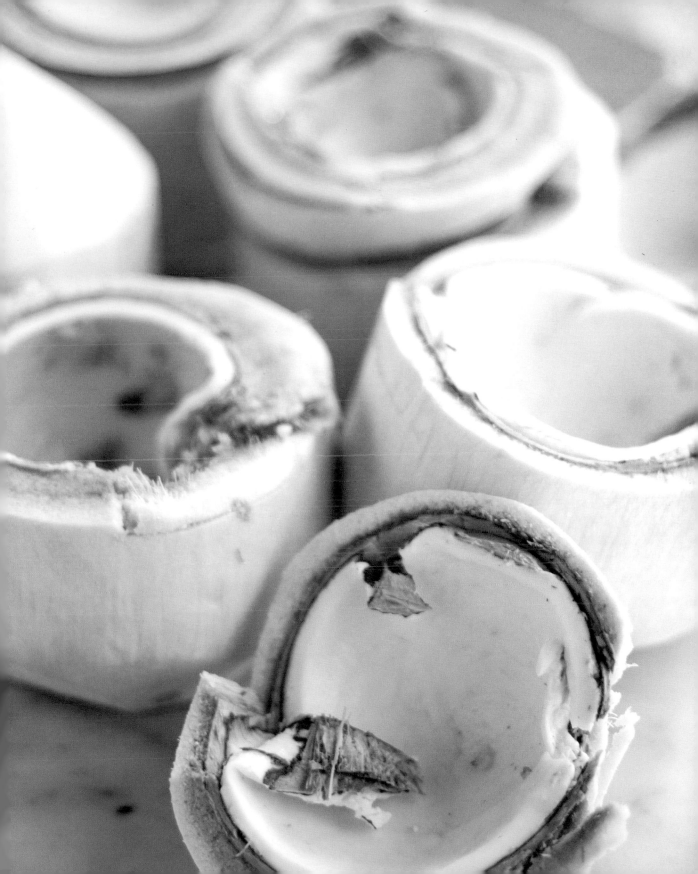

Piña Colada

You can taste the tropics in this shake. It's like an instant vacation.

> "This is one of my favorite shakes. And it becomes even more of a favorite when I make a particularly happy variation with sake (page 331)." —SM

1 cup coconut meat
1 ¹/₂ cups coconut water
3 cups diced pineapple
3 tablespoons agave nectar or 2 packets stevia
1 tablespoon coconut butter
Squeeze of lime juice
2 teaspoons vanilla extract
Pinch of sea salt

In a blender, puree all ingredients until smooth.

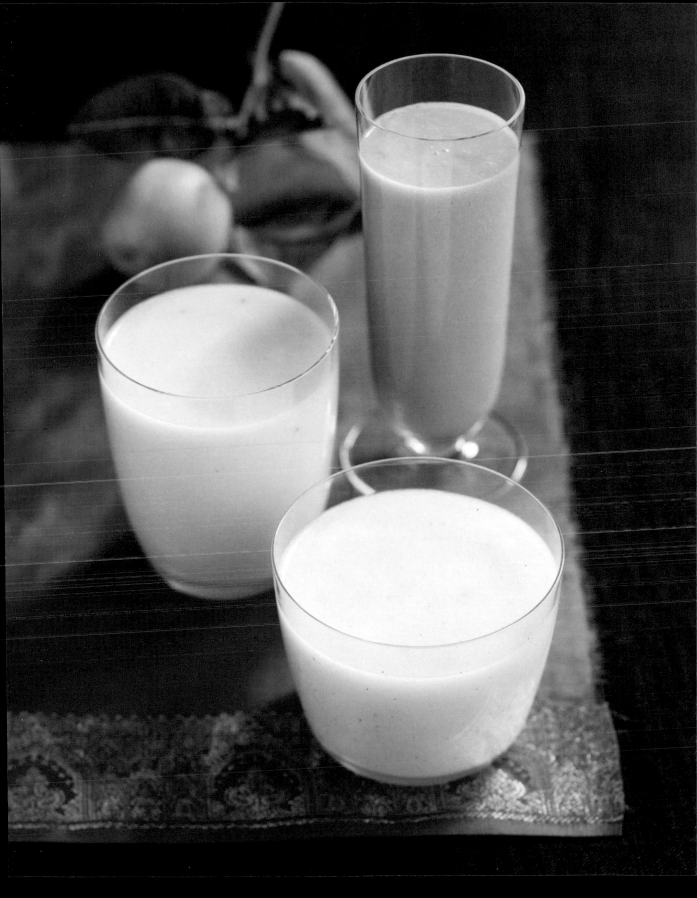

Creamy Coconut Shake

SERVES 2 TO 4

The medium chain fatty acids in coconut are more likely to be used for energy and less likely to be stored as fat, compared to other fats. It has powerful antibacterial and antiviral properties and is particularly good for boosting immunity. It's pure fuel for your body that tastes like an indulgence.

If you can get fresh, organic vanilla beans, use the seeds of one half bean here instead of the extract. The vanilla flavor is better and the specks look good in the pure white liquid.

> "We can't decide if we love this shake more because of how good it tastes or because of how good it is for you." —MK

2 cups coconut meat
3 cups coconut water
¹/₄ cup agave nectar or 3 packets stevia
1 tablespoon lime juice
2 teaspoons vanilla extract
Pinch of sea salt

In a blender, puree all ingredients until smooth.

Avocolada

Avocados originally hail from Guatemala and have since been adapted to amenable climates all over South- and Central America, the southeast and southwest United States, the Caribbean, and Asia. They are an important fruit in the raw food diet. Rich in beneficial oil, the avocado is replete with minerals that are great for the skin and hair. The flavor of this tropical fruit, which has hundreds of varieties, can range from sweet to almost garlicky, and the texture from rich and smooth to more watery and chunky. The sweet and creamy Haas avocado, which is harvested in California year-round, is the most widely available variety and best to use in these recipes.

> Nick Ross, a longtime server at our restaurant, loves to wander into the juice bar and concoct tasty and unusual shakes that are so good, we usually end up putting them on the menu. A little avocado in smoothies is great (just don't add too much or you'll think you're drinking guacamole). —SM

1 ripe avocado, peeled and pitted
3 cups diced pineapple
2 cups coconut water
3 tablespoons agave nectar or 2 packets stevia
3 tablespoons lime juice
1 tablespoon coconut butter (optional)
2 teaspoons vanilla extract
Pinch of sea salt

In a blender, puree all ingredients until smooth.

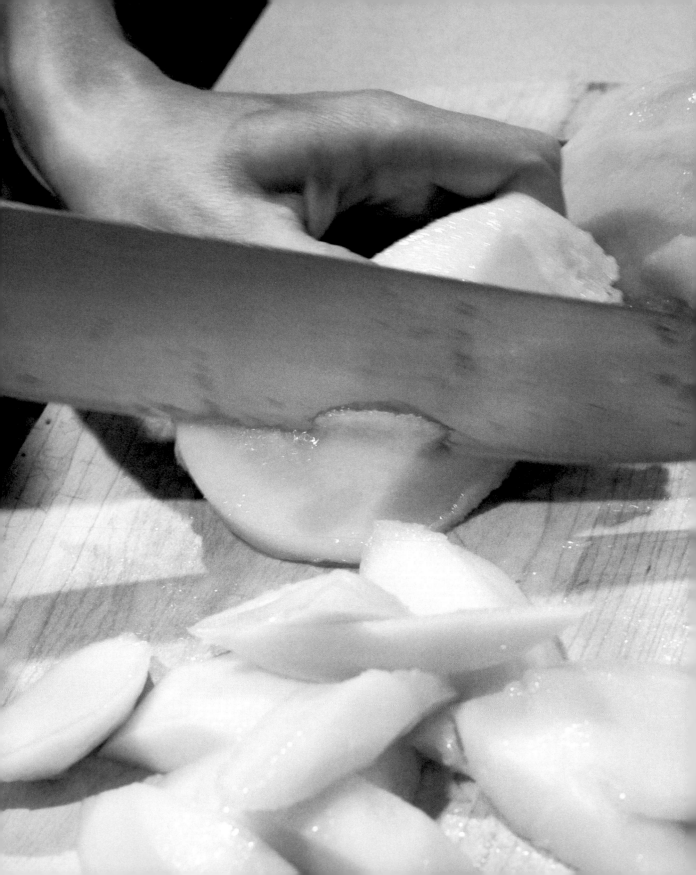

Mango Shake

SERVES 2 TO 4

The world's most popular fruit, mangos have inspired poets, chefs, and gods, and as such are the stuff of legends. From 400 to 1,000 varieties grow in tropical and subtropical climates all over the globe. They can weigh anywhere from a few ounces to more than 2 pounds, and when picked ripe are so juicy that most people eat them while in a pool or bathtub (now that's raw food at its best!). Both green and ripe mangos are savored for their accessibility and versatility, and are especially important in Asian, Caribbean, and Central Mexican cuisines.

Most of the mangos you see in North American markets during the winter hail from Mexico and Central America, where they were picked too young and stored in refrigerated warehouses until the natural season ended. Mangos are a good lesson in why we should always eat seasonally. If you've ever had a perfectly blushed Haden, sun-warm and plucked from a giving tree (ripe mangos offer no resistance when they're picked, though green ones will), then you know what we mean. From May to October, look for mangos that have been shipped from Florida and the Caribbean, or better yet, make friends with someone who has a tree. After all, that's what we did (our coauthor, who lives in Miami, has fourteen trees, and she promises to share).

> **If you ever see Thai mangos in the market, scoop them up. They are flatter with a yellow skin and somewhat stringy flesh, and the flavor is even more exotic and intoxicating than the more common mangos. They are a bit harder to work with, but it's worth it.** —MK

3 cups diced mango
2 cups coconut water
3 tablespoons agave nectar or 2 packets stevia

2 teaspoons vanilla extract
Squeeze of lime juice
Pinch of sea salt

In a blender, puree all ingredients until smooth.

Super Green Powder

These green powders are gaining in popularity as a "superfood." Find one that is made from 100 percent raw, organic, and/or wildcrafted vegetables and algaes, including wheatgrass, barley grass, spirulina, and others. They also usually contain probiotics to implant beneficial bacteria in the intestines. We recommend Nature's First Food and Pure Synergy (see Sources, page 362). Super green food powders taste best in fruit-based shakes, particularly those with berries, or in fruit juices. Very often, when we make fruit shakes, we'll pour most of it into our glasses, leaving a small amount in the blender cup. Then we'll add a full tablespoon of green powder to the blender, as well as any other supplement that has a funny taste, such as maca powder. We drink the small quantity of funny tasting shake first and then have our larger, still-fruity-flavored and pretty-colored shakes left to enjoy!

Enzyme Boost

Papayas contain a lot of enzymes that are terrific for your skin (you can even buy papaya enzyme supplements in health food stores). This is why you see many papaya-based skin care products on the market—although you don't have to buy any of them. Simply mash up a bit of fresh papaya (the less ripe ones contain more enzymes) and put it on your face like a mask until it dries, then rinse off. Papayas are a cleansing fruit and contain a large amount of calcium, vitamin A, and vitamin C.

The smaller Hawaiian papayas, sometimes called "strawberry papayas," have a fruitier flavor. But because they are more delicate than the larger Mexican papayas, they are more labor intensive to peel and seed. We like to eat the smaller, tastier papayas whole and use the larger ones for shakes.

Pineapples also contain a large quantity of enzymes, which are mostly concentrated around the core. Its slightly acidic and tart flavors balance the papaya, which can be ultrasweet, especially when very ripe.

> Matthew and I are big fans of the papaya mask, which we like to do when making this shake. Just don't forget you have it on, as we occasionally do and then wonder why our FedEx guy looks at us so strangely when we answer the door. —SM

2 cups diced pineapple
2 cups diced papaya, peeled and seeded
1¹/₂ cups coconut water
3 tablespoons agave nectar or 2 packets stevia

2 teaspoons vanilla extract
Squeeze of lime juice
Pinch of sea salt

In a blender, blend all of the ingredients until smooth.

Blue Sunset

SERVES 2 TO 4

Blueberries are hailed as a superfood for their abundant antioxidants; even popular science has come to realize the boost a body gets from blueberries. We're especially partial to the tiny, intensely flavored, wild Maine blueberries, but these can be difficult to find outside the state (and, of course, off-season). Either wild or the more common cultivated blueberries can be frozen to give shakes an icy quality.

> "Melvin, the best juicer in New York, who also happens to run our own juice bar for us at night, made me this shake one day. The colors are so pretty that everyone wants one when they see it." —SM

2 cups pineapple chunks
1 small, ripe banana or 1 cup frozen diced banana
1 cup diced mango
1¹/₂ cups Brazil nut milk or macadamia milk (see pages 52 and 62), or coconut water
3 tablespoons agave nectar or 2 packets stevia
2 teaspoons vanilla extract
Pinch of sea salt
1 cup blueberries

In a blender, puree all ingredients except blueberries until smooth. Pour out about half of the mixture into serving glasses, filling each glass halfway. Add the blueberries to the remaining shake in the blender and blend until smooth. Gently pour the remaining blueberry shake over the pineapple-mango shake. Note: Pouring the mixture over the back of a spoon (a bartender's technique) helps keep the two layers separate.

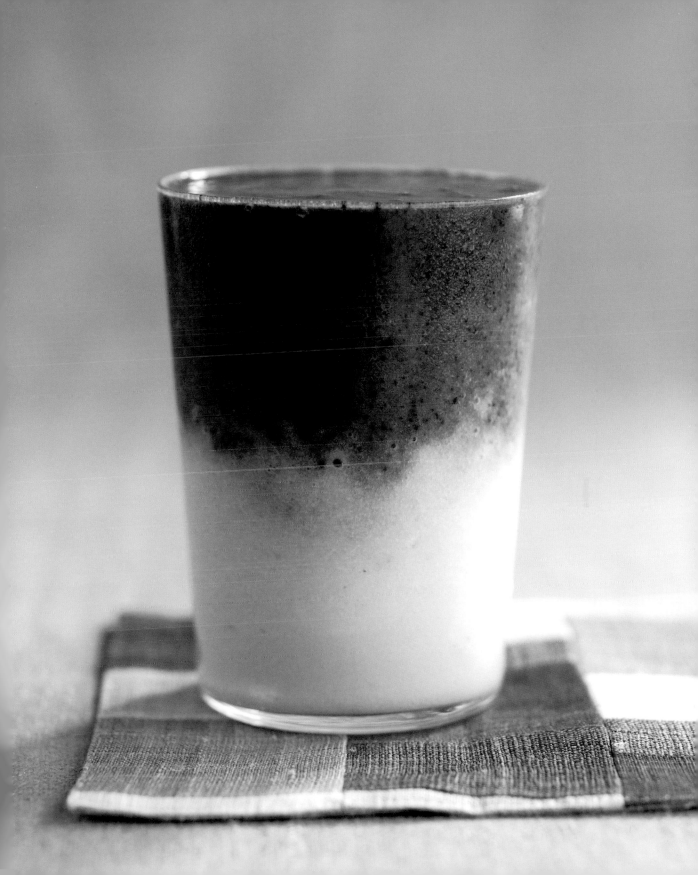

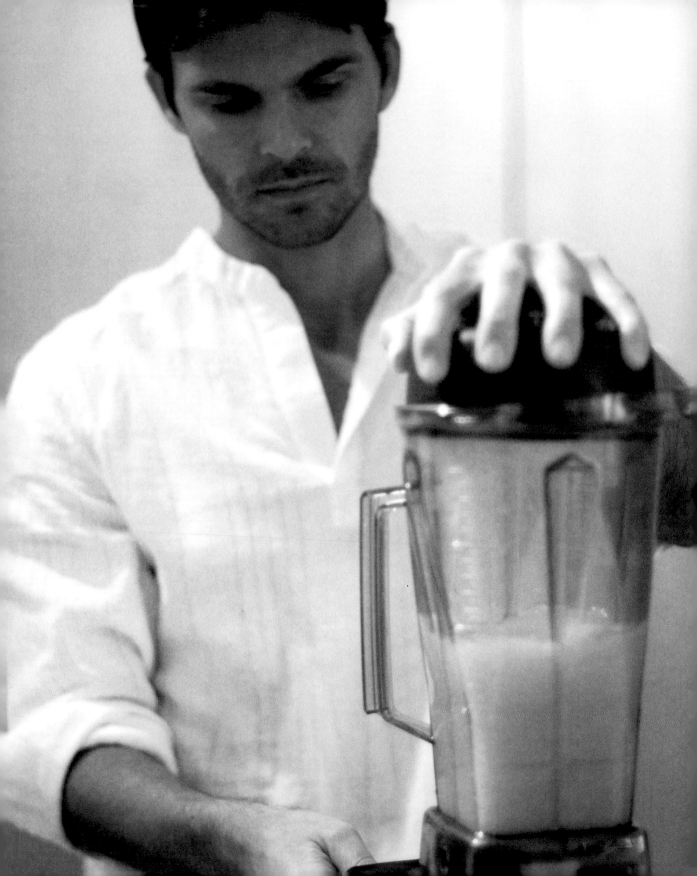

Bunny Spice

Carrot juice is a great source of beta-carotene (as everyone knows by now), and a powerful antioxidant. However, carrots are also hybridized and much sweeter than wild carrots would be, and so we avoid consuming too many of them. Fresh ginger is great for digestion or settling an upset stomach, and it improves circulation.

> "This is another Nick Ross creation . . . when he gave it to me I had to drink half of it before I could place the flavors—it's so good, and yet unexpected to have carrot in a creamy sweet shake." —SM

1 cup carrot-ginger juice (run carrots through the juicer with a thumb-size knob of fresh gingerroot)
1 cup almond milk or Brazil nut milk (see pages 57 and 52)
2 cups frozen diced banana
Pinch of ground cinnamon

In a blender, puree all ingredients until smooth.

Tocotrienols

"Tocos," as we call them, are a potent source of vitamin E extracted from the husk of rice bran. Tocos also contain over 100 known antioxidants as well as essential fatty acids, vitamins, minerals, and enzymes that help protect the body from the formation of free radicals and degenerative disease. Tocos are really good for your skin, too—by the time you read this, they'll be the next buzz word in facial creams, the way lycopene and white tea extract have been recently. Tocos have a very mild malted flavor that is slightly sweet, and they go well in any creamy shake. Add 1 heaping tablespoon per serving. As a fluffy, crystalline powder, it can be a great ingredient in desserts as well, but is very expensive, so we don't use it too often in that way. See Sources, page 362 for where to buy it.

Ground Flaxseed

Containing rich, healthy fatty acids (omega-3, omega-6, and omega-9) that are needed for the human body to function, ground flaxseed is a great supplement (and very affordable). It also provides soluble fiber and is high in lignans, which are hormone-like substances that are known to balance hormone levels in the body. Place brown or golden flaxseeds in a coffee or spice grinder to pulverize and add a tablespoon or so to any shake, but keep in mind it will add a bit of flavor and color, so it works best in darker, fruit and berry shakes.

Peruvian Maca

This is a powdered supplement that comes from the Peruvian maca root. It contains amino acids, complex carbohydrates, vitamins B_1, B_2, B_{12}, C, and E and minerals, including calcium, phosphorus, zinc, magnesium, and iron. Among many other purported benefits, it is said to be excellent for balancing hormones, building muscle, enhancing stamina, and increasing fertility. Maca tastes a bit funny, almost like powdered sweet potato. It goes best in shakes with plenty of banana or other strong flavors. If you don't love the taste, you can also find the powder in capsule form. See Sources, page 360 for where to buy it.

Cinnamon Banana Shake

SERVES 2 TO 4

> " I make this and the Chocolate Banana Shake (page 85) for Matthew all the time when he's hungry and we don't have fresh ingredients in the house. We always have frozen bananas in the freezer, and almond butter in the fridge to stand in for fresh nut milk. " —SM

3 cups frozen diced banana
2 cups Brazil nut milk or almond milk (pages 52 and 57) or try the 30-Second Nut Milk, page 58)
3 tablespoons agave nectar or 2 packets stevia
1 teaspoon vanilla extract
$1/2$ teaspoon ground cinnamon
Pinch of sea salt

In a blender, puree all ingredients until smooth and creamy.

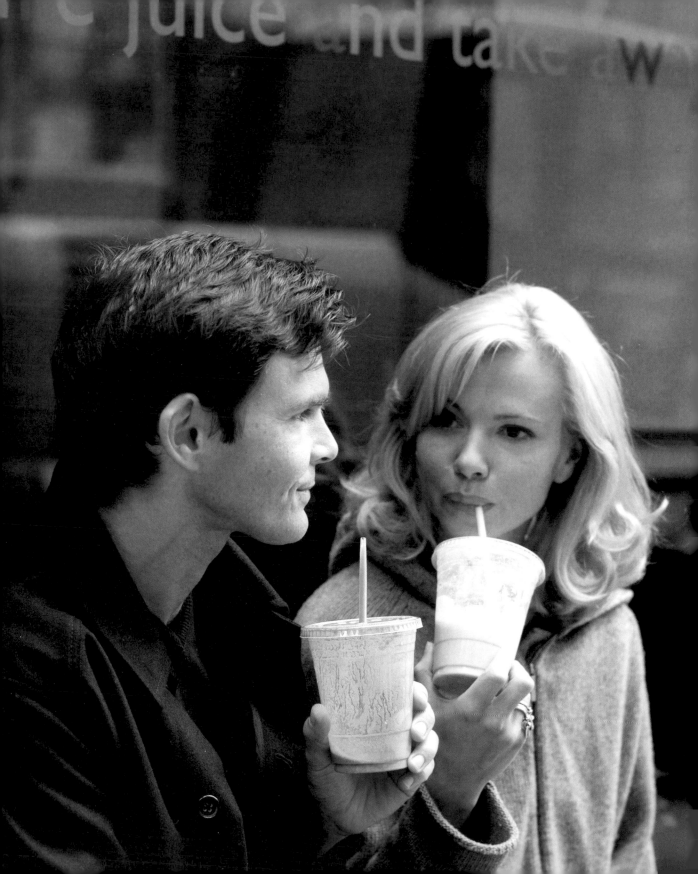

Chocolate Banana Shake

SERVES 2 TO 4

Use either organic cocoa powder or raw carob powder in this shake (or a combination of both). Carob powder comes from the pods of carob trees that grow in the Mediterranean. Carob does not contain any of the stimulants that are found in cocoa and it's high in calcium. We feel carob is hugely underappreciated, but try it in this shake and you might just prefer it to chocolate.

> **If the bananas are ripe when they are frozen, and frozen when they are added to this shake, it is nearly impossible for anyone to fault it. It is rich, creamy, chocolatey, and satisfying. And I can easily drink the whole recipe!** —MK

3 cups frozen diced banana
2 cups Brazil nut or almond milk (see pages 52 and 57), or 30-Second Nut Milk (page 58)
1/4 cup agave nectar or 2 packets stevia
1 teaspoon vanilla extract
2 heaping tablespoons organic cocoa powder or carob powder
Pinch of sea salt

In a blender, puree all ingredients until smooth and creamy.

Bee Protein

This shake is *full* of good stuff! The hemp provides a hefty dose of protein along with all the essential amino acids; the almond butter adds more protein along with vitamin E, magnesium, folic acid; and the bee pollen gives still more high quality protein, essential amino acids, and enzymes. Raw honey is rich in B-complex vitamins; vitamins C, D, and E; and is a great source of the enzyme amylase, which helps to break down sugars. Bananas add potassium, while mangos are full of vitamin A and are one of the richest sources of carotenoids, which help ward off colds and reduce the risk of cancer and heart disease.

> We came up with this shake to put on the menu at a juice bar in a big gym in Manhattan. It's for all the meatheads who want 'protein shakes' with 'protein powders'— this is our nutritionally superior and totally all-natural and tasty alternative. —SM

2 heaping tablespoons almond butter

2 cups coconut water, or filtered water

1 cup diced mango

1 cup frozen diced banana

1 heaping tablespoon hemp protein (see Sources, page 359)

1 tablespoon bee pollen (see Sources, page 358)

2 heaping tablespoons raw honey

2 teaspoons vanilla extract

Pinch of sea salt

In a blender, puree all ingredients until smooth and creamy.

Bee Pollen

Bee pollen is granulated pollen gathered by the bees and is one of nature's most complete, nutritious foods. About 40 percent protein, half of which is free amino acids, bee pollen supplies humans with almost every essential element we need to survive. It is also markedly high in folic acid, vitamins, and nucleic acids, and is thought to help cure chronic digestive and autoimmune diseases. And women, listen up: Not only has bee pollen been tapped to stimulate the production of eggs from ovaries, it also plays a role in preventing and treating such cancers as breast and uterine. In this case, a spoonful of honey just might save your life. See Sources, page 358, for where to buy it.

> "I used to blend a tablespoon of bee pollen into our fruit-based shakes, but it gave them a bit of a funny pasty taste that I didn't love. However, now I've really grown to like the flavor of bee pollen eaten on its own, so I often sprinkle it on top of our shakes and eat it with a spoon." —SM

Hemp Protein

Made from hemp seeds, this supplement has a 45 percent protein content. Adding raw organic hemp protein powder to vegan foods is a significant way to increase protein intake. (However, you may want to see the textbox on page 123 for an explanation of why we don't need to be as obsessed about getting enough protein as many people are!) As the powder has a nutty flavor, it's not a match for all foods, milks, or shakes. Hemp protein has no saturated fats or cholesterol, and is safe for diabetics and hypoglycemics. Always store hemp powder in the refrigerator to retain freshness. See Sources, page 359, for where to buy it.

Fig and Grape Cleansing Shake

SERVES 2 TO 4

Grapes are among the most cleansing fruits, full of vitamins and minerals. Try to find organic grapes *with* seeds—the seeds contain powerful antioxidants (to fight those pesky free radicals) and essential fatty oils (excellent for skin and hair—note the recent trend in expensive beauty products to include grapeseed oils and extract). The skins also contain a substance called resveratrol that is known to inhibit cancer growth and protect against coronary heart disease. There is even a book called *The Grape Cure* written by Johanna Brandt in the 1930s, who claimed to have healed her stomach cancer with grapes. As for figs, they are incredibly high in calcium and are a good natural laxative, with tiny seeds and a substance called mucin to help clean toxins and mucus out of the system. Dr. Arnold Ehret, who wrote so entertainingly about natural foods and fasting in the 1920s, called figs one of his top three "mucus-dissolving" foods.

> Aesthetically, it's nice to use green grapes with pale-colored Calimyrna figs for a lighter shake and red grapes with black mission figs for a dark shake, although it really doesn't matter if you mix it up. The recipe calls for dried figs, because they are more readily available year-round, but use fresh if you can get them—just reduce the amount of water by about half. —MK

4 cups green or red grapes
1 cup dried Calimyrna or black mission figs, hard stems removed
1 cup cold filtered water

$^1/_2$ teaspoon vanilla extract
$^1/_8$ teaspoon ground star anise (or cinnamon)
Pinch of sea salt
2 cups ice cubes

In a Vita-Mix or high-speed blender, add grapes and puree at high speed until smooth. If using seeded grapes, blend until seeds are thoroughly pureed. Add the figs, water, vanilla, star anise, and salt and blend at high speed until completely smooth. Add ice cubes and blend until just smooth.

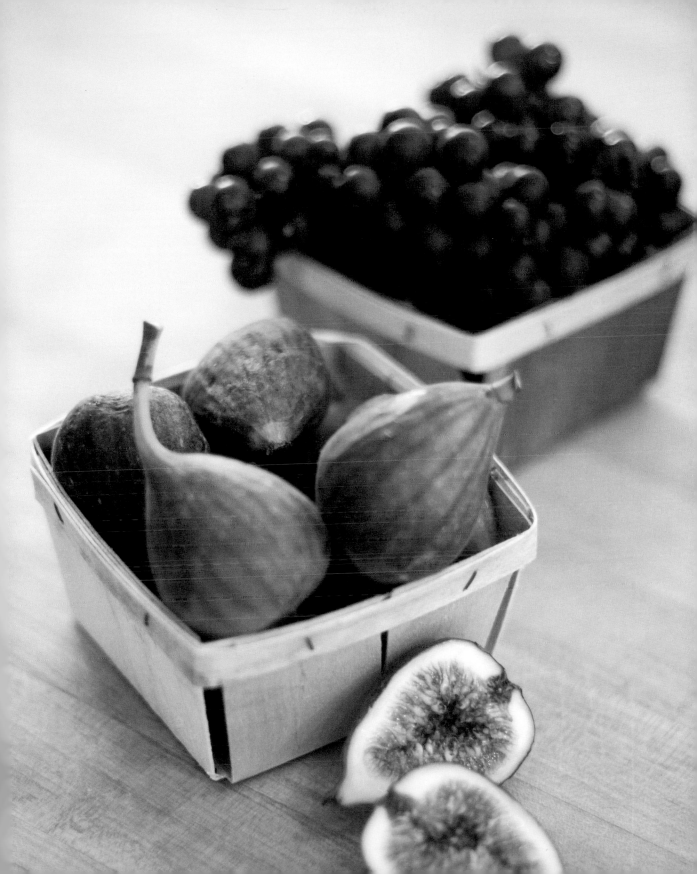

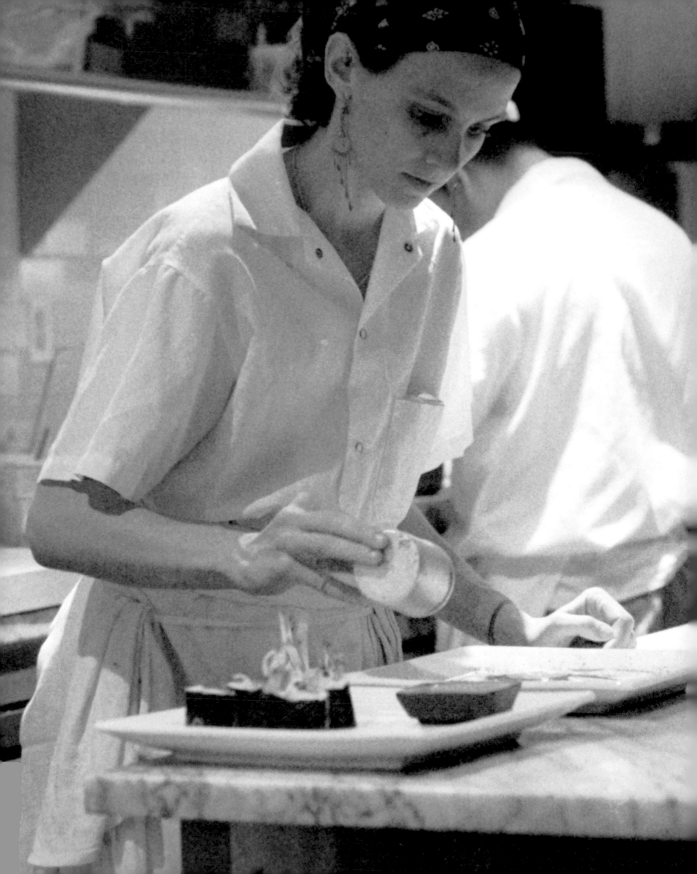

Salt

Salt is not the enemy. It is necessary for our brain function, and for balancing our systems. When combined with the right foods, salt optimizes flavor. Commercial table salt, however, is the proverbial friend that might as well be an enemy. Flash-dried at scorching temperatures and chemically bleached, table salt, which is often reinforced with iodine, just doesn't do anything for you—in fact, it's *bad* for you. Ditto rock or kosher salt, which is mined from dried-out beds where water used to be. Sea salt, skimmed from the tops of stationary tidal pools and dried in the sun, is moist, flaky crystals with minerals in every shard. For our purposes, Celtic sea salt—hand-harvested and dried slowly under the Brittany sun—is among the most nutritious, containing more than 80 minerals, including calcium.

Another type of salt recently getting a buzz among raw foodies and health-minded people is Himalayan Crystal Salt (see Sources, page 361), considered a truly precious, holistic salt. *Water and Salt—The Essence of Life*, a book by Dr. Barbara Hendel, M.D. and biophysicist Peter Fierra, describes the healing powers of this salt, harvested from the Himalayan Mountains. We get ours from David Kaplan, known around our place as "The Salt Guy," as in, "Sarma, there's a guy here to speak to you about *salt*?" We sell his salt in our store, and use it at the restaurant and at home. To quote straight from the box, "[The] natural method of mining assures that the original vibration pattern, the inherent stored information within the crystals, their essential elements, remain fully intact and vital. In this natural, holistic form the salt is of supreme bioenergetic quality." Neither of us is quite sure what "bioenergetic qualities" are, but the salt really tastes amazing.

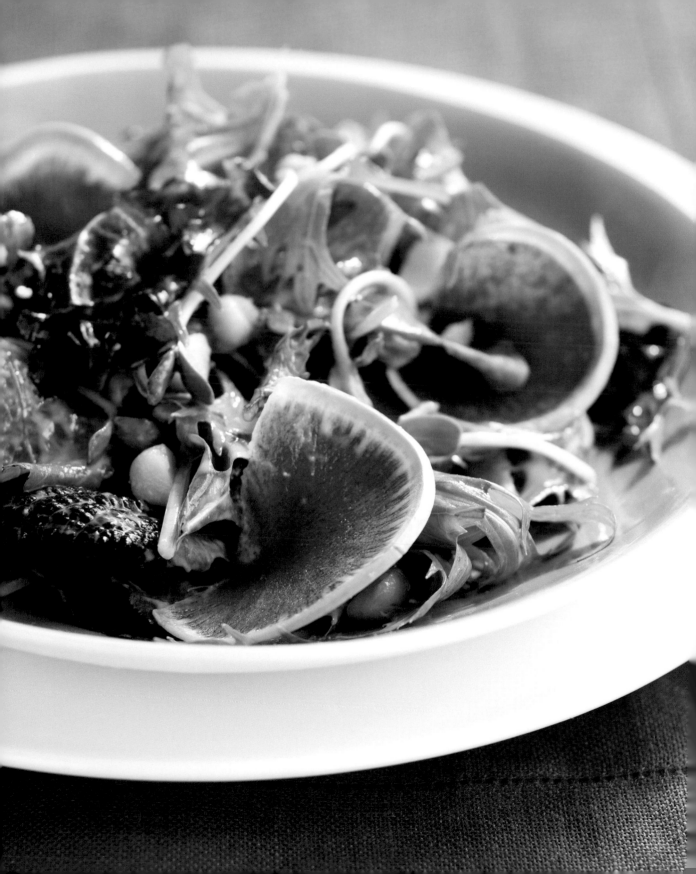

SALADS

Popularized by Popeye, greens (dark leafy ones in particular) are the foods that make us big and strong. Perhaps more significantly, the salads we can make out of these greens, plus related garnishes and dressings, are simply the most satisfying meals that one can eat. We actually felt this way long before we ever discovered the raw food lifestyle.

Very often we made salads as a main dish when cooking for ourselves. If not, we would generally have one *with* our meals, which we have since learned is the most important thing you can do if you are going to eat cooked foods, meat and fish in particular. Greens help you properly digest other foods.

We think salads are a great opportunity for creativity, because you can easily combine many ingredients, and because you can unite so many varying textures and flavors and get them all in one bite. A large bowl filled with crispy lettuces, smoky dulse, hemp seeds, creamy avocado, red pepper macadamia cheese, fresh herbs, citrus, and olive oil is satiating beyond belief to both the palate and the appetite.

Constructing salads is easy, but keep in mind that some factors do apply to the making of a great salad. Think of them as vegetable sundaes—they're never wrong if you like the results, but they still follow a basic pattern.

First, we always make sure to find the best ingredients that are available to us. Begin by following the seasons and learn what fresh products you will have plenty of access to and when. In general, the darker the greens, the more packed with vitamins they are. We like to mix heartier varieties (spinach, baby chard, kale) with spicy or just-bitter greens (mustard, arugula, frisee, watercress) and other lighter, softer lettuces (baby romaine, red oak, lolla rosa, and bibb). When available, microgreens are also a great addition (see page 113). The chlorophyll-rife greens form the basis of most of our salads, although some of our recipes highlight other seasonal ingredients of superior quality—a fennel-based salad, for example, can be incredible with ruby red grapefruit and mint.

When we are making our salads both at home and at the restaurant, we always try to balance the flavors and textures: leveling acidity from citrus with oils; playing off something creamy like avocados with something crunchy like nuts; adding a sweet element with fresh or dried fruit to counter bitter lettuces. The best example of this is Our Favorite Filling Salad on page 110.

Many of the recipes for dressings in this chapter make more than you actually need for a salad for 4 or even 6, but it's not always convenient to blend very small quantities—it's generally difficult to blend anything less than a cup of liquid. Fortunately, most of these dressings keep at least 2 or 3 days in the refrigerator, so save the leftovers for future salads or just for dipping vegetables.

Greenmarket Salad

with macadamia nuts and creamy citrus dressing

SERVES 4

In general, greenmarkets are another name for farmer's markets. These are the best places to get your greens, as the growers usually pick, clip, or snip (with scissors) the greens the night before or even the morning of the event. For the same reasons, green-markets are also ideal for purchasing sprouts. At the Union Square Greenmarket in New York City, Stuart, "the wheatgrass guy" (known for growing the sweetest wheatgrass around), also has trays of fresh sunflower sprouts, which he cuts for you on the spot when you buy them. These are so much more deliciously crisp than the prepackaged kind that you sometimes find in stores, which are more often than not beginning to get slimy. The fresh sprouts keep very well in the refrigerator, with the bag propped open a bit to give them some air. If purchased very fresh, they can last up to a week, although they are best to eat within a few days.

This dressing is so yummy, you could almost drink it. —SM

For the dressing:

1 small avocado, peeled and pitted
1 cup orange juice
$^1/_4$ cup plus 2 tablespoons lime juice
1 handful cilantro
1 green onion, white and 1 inch of green, coarsely chopped
1 tablespoon chopped shallot
$^1/_2$ small jalapeño
$^1/_2$ teaspoon sea salt
$^1/_2$ cup olive oil
Freshly ground black pepper

In a blender, add the avocado, orange and lime juices, cilantro, green onion, shallot, jalapeño, and salt and blend until smooth. With the blender running, slowly pour in the olive oil, allowing it to emulsify for a thick, creamy consistency. Season to taste with pepper.

Makes 2$^1/_2$ cups

For the salad:

1 large bowlful mixed fresh salad greens
1 large handful sunflower sprouts (optional)
2 watermelon radishes (or other variety), trimmed and sliced thin on a mandoline
$^1/_2$ cup raw macadamia nuts, coarsely chopped
1 teaspoon macadamia nut oil or other cold-pressed oil
Pinch of coarse sea salt
Freshly ground black pepper

1 In a large bowl, gently toss the salad greens, sprouts (if using), and most of the radishes (reserving some for garnish) with enough of the dressing to generously coat the leaves. You will have leftover dressing—store it in the refrigerator for 2 to 3 days.

2 In a small bowl, toss the nuts with the oil and salt. Divide the greens among 4 plates or bowls. Sprinkle with the nuts and garnish with the remaining radish slices. Add pepper to taste.

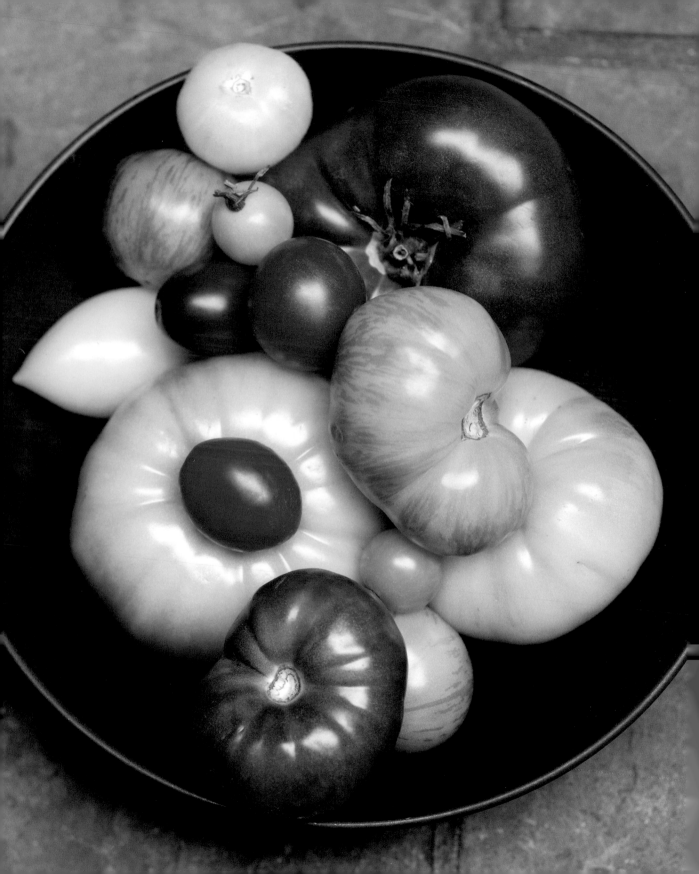

Going Organic: It Takes a Community

Unless you actually like the idea of consuming chemicals with your corn and beans, you are probably pretty clear on why eating pesticide-free heirloom, wild, and sustainably raised fruits, nuts, grains, and vegetables is not just a choice but a responsibility. Simply put, pesticides are poison. How can they not affect our nervous systems? The damage may not be as immediate or severe as a roach flopping over on its back and seizing after being sprayed, but over time the consequences of eating chemically tainted food could be far-reaching.

Pesticides are not the only compelling reason to go organic. As Gabriel Cousens, M.D., writes in his book *Rainbow Green Live-Food Cuisine*, "For those interested in health, what we are looking at is an unsavory situation. We are faced with commercially grown foods, irradiated foods, genetically engineered foods, and government authorities who are choosing, in essence, to make it very difficult to discern whether something has been irradiated or genetically modified."

Cousens encourages the consumer to buy organic with his claim that "foods produced by organic farming methods exhibit improved vitamin and mineral nutrition, as well as superior taste, shelf-life, and phytochemical and antioxidant content." In fact, government studies show that the rate of nutrition in conventionally farmed food has steadily declined since the 1940s, and practices such as fertilization and genetic interference are being held to blame.

We don't need to overintellectualize it, either. Even monkeys know the difference between organic and nonorganic foods. As reported in the May/June 2003 issue of the *Well Being Journal*, the tapirs and chimpanzees at the Copenhagen Zoo, who were introduced to organic foods in 2002, reject nonorganic bananas in favor of those naturally grown when both are left in their cages. They'll even eat the whole organic banana, skin and all. But when it comes to the conventional fruit, if that's all that's available in their cages, they'll actually peel the fruit first and discard the skin. Perhaps they can smell the gases that are often used to ripen bananas that have been picked green. Whatever the reason for it, if it makes sense to a monkey, why doesn't it make sense to us?

Money, that's why. The biggest complaint the average consumer has about organic foods is the expense. And it's true, organic fruits and vegetables often have higher price tags.

It's a vicious cycle: costs are high because demand and production are low. To get our organic grocery bill down, we have to spend more, at least temporarily. Once we begin to clamor for nonconventionally farmed produce on a wide-scale basis, the market will respond.

You also don't have to resort to the gas-ripened, mass-produced, hothouse tomato over the more exclusive Brandywine or Green Zebra just because you're short on money or time. An alternative is to rely on your community—specifically, Community-Supported Agriculture (CSA).

CSA is based on a system called *teikei* (meaning "partnership") that was developed by a cooperative of Japanese women who were tired of using imported products and wanted "to put the farmer's face to the food." The concept spread to Europe and then to North America, where Jan Vander Tuin, who ran a CSA in Switzerland, introduced the idea to Robyn Van En of Indian Line Farm in 1984. Today there are more than 1,000 CSAs across the country.

An enticing alternative to the anonymous shopping we do at high-end health food supermarket, the CSA process is similar to investing in the stock market. Before the planting season begins, the consumer buys a prix-fixe "share" in the harvest that will be brought in by a farm or a farm collective. In return, the consumer receives a box of fruit and vegetables—whatever happens to be ripe—on a set day every week.

Many of the farms that participate in CSA programs are small, family-run concerns that tend to be, if not certified organic (in some states it can take five years to become certified), at least pesticide-free and sustainable. Participating is a gamble, because it could be a drought year or an entire crop could be washed away in floods. But the farmers generally plant a wide variety so that if one crop doesn't take, it's not a disaster. And the benefits of participating in a CSA are as multipronged as a fork: the vine-and tree-ripe produce tastes better; overall the items cost less; food is kept locally and eaten seasonally, cutting down on fossil fuel consumption and the myth that mangos bloom year-round; and the "surprise" factor of the contents of the box keeps it interesting.

If you suspect a CSA might exist quite literally in your own backyard, the Robyn Van En Center (www.csacenter.org) should be your first research stop.

Arugula Salad

with pear, spiced pumpkin seeds, and meyer lemon dressing

The Meyer lemon, imported in 1908 from China, is a lot sweeter, juicier, and bigger than the Eureka or Lisbon lemon you find in the typical grocery store. The Meyer lemon tree typically has two seasons per year, and its pith and seeds are antiseptic, antimicrobial, and odor-alleviating—try rubbing them under your arms instead of using environment-harming aerosol deodorant sprays (no, we're not kidding). Meyer lemons are fairly easy to find during the season (November, December, and January in most areas) in the warmer climates, where citrus is an important crop, and in large metropolises such as New York, though they are hard to locate elsewhere. Fortunately, there are online sources as well as easy-care container trees that are great for producing indoor crops in cold climates, so you can actually grow your own lemons! (see Sources, page 360)

Make sure to keep some of the white pith on when you cut the lemons. Limonene, which is found in the pith, has been recognized as a potent anticancer nutrient.

Don't worry if Meyer lemons are out of season or if you can't find them locally. You can very easily use regular lemons, but you will probably want to add a bit more honey to balance out the tartness. We do this at the restaurant.

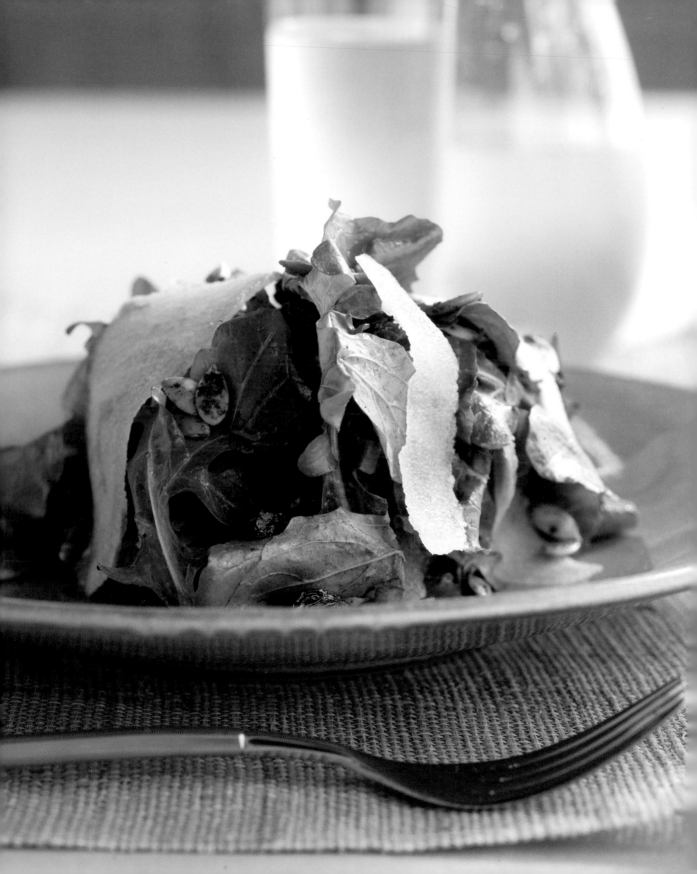

For the dressing:

4 whole Meyer lemons
2 tablespoons raw honey
1/3 cup extra-virgin olive oil
1/4 teaspoon sea salt
Freshly ground black pepper

With a sharp paring knife, cut away the ends and the outer peel of the lemons, leaving some of the white pith. Cut the lemons in halves or quarters and add to the blender with the honey. Blend on high speed for about a minute to fully break up the seeds and pith. With the blender running on medium speed, slowly pour in the olive oil. Season with the sea salt and pepper to taste.

Makes 1 cup

For the salad:

1 pound washed arugula leaves
1 pear, cut into shavings with a peeler
1/2 cup Candied Pumpkin Seeds (page 288)
1/2 cup dried cherries or cranberries

In a large mixing bowl, gently toss the greens and pear with enough dressing to generously coat. Divide among serving plates and sprinkle with the pumpkin seeds and dried cherries.

Sea Vegetable Salad
with pickled sour cherries
and sweet miso dressing

SERVES 4

This dressing is good with all kinds of salads, particularly a big salad of mixed sprouts. We find that really flavorful dressings go well with sea vegetables, particularly if you have not become accustomed to eating them yet.

Most packaged varieties of sea vegetables come in 2-ounce packages, and here we call for about half a package of each variety, which is about the equivalent of one large handful each.

One of our sous-chefs at the restaurant, Louisa, came up with this salad. Keep in mind that you don't have to follow this recipe exactly if you want to keep things simple; you can add chopped greens or sunflower sprouts to lighten it up a bit in place of the julienned vegetables. The pickled sour cherries are a nice tart element, but if fresh cherries are not in season, pickle some sliced plums instead, substituting about one thin slice per plump cherry. Or forget the pickling and just use fresh cherries or plums—the salad is great that way as well.　—MK

For the pickled cherries:

1 cup sour cherries, pitted and halved
$^1/_2$ cup vinegar, preferably raw apple cider vinegar
3 tablespoons agave nectar

In a small bowl, add the cherries, vinegar, and agave nectar and stir to combine well. Let it sit for at least half an hour. Drain the cherries and set aside.

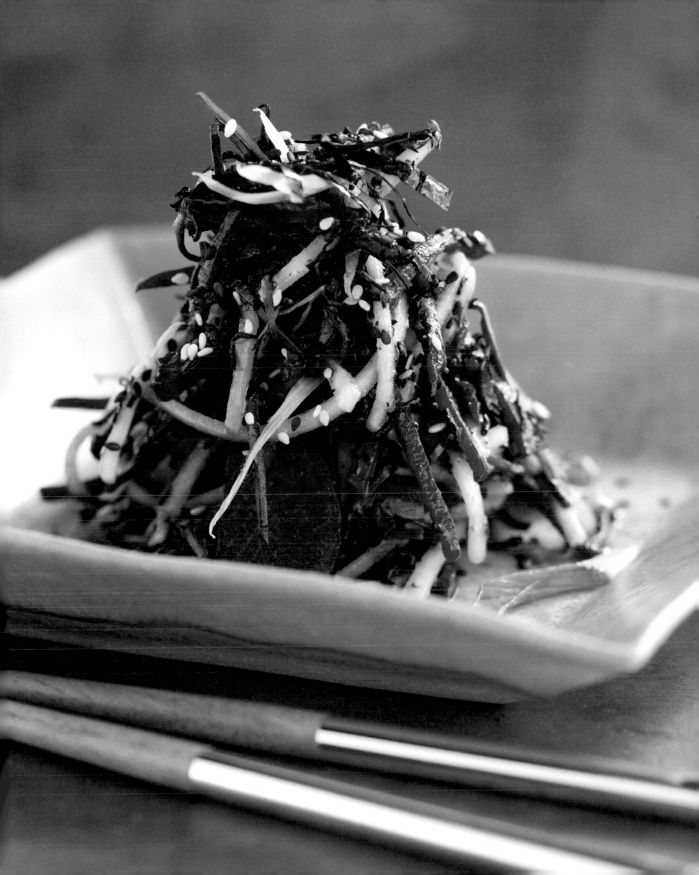

For the sweet miso dressing

½ cup white miso

⅓ cup agave nectar

½ cup mirin

¼ cup sesame oil

¼ cup lemon juice

¼ cup chopped ginger

In a blender, blend all ingredients until smooth. Store the leftover dressing in the refrigerator for 3 to 4 days. Makes about 2 cups.

For the salad:

1 ounce dried wakame

1 ounce dried hijiki

1 ounce dried arame

1 large cucumber, peeled, seeded, and
    julienned

2 large beets, peeled and julienned

1 medium daikon radish, peeled and julienned

1 green onion, white and 1 inch of green,
    very thinly sliced on a bias

2 tablespoons black sesame seeds

2 tablespoons white sesame seeds

½ sheet dry nori, cut in half, stacked,
    and cut into thin strips (optional)

1. In separate bowls, soak the sea vegetables in water until soft and pliable. The arame softens very quickly, so you will want to drain off the water after 5 to 10 minutes. The hijiki and wakame take at least 20 minutes. But try not to let any of the sea vegetables soak too long. They should be soft, but not waterlogged (think al dente pasta).

2. Drain the sea vegetables and, using your hands, squeeze out as much of the water as possible. This is important so the sea vegetables do not get mushy. Roughly chop the wakame into smaller, more manageable pieces. Place the sea vegetables in a large bowl and add the cucumber, beets, radish, and pickled cherries.

3. If you are making this ahead of time, do not add the dressing until ready to serve. Add about half the dressing to the vegetables and toss gently to combine. Add more dressing according to taste. Divide among 4 serving dishes, and sprinkle with the green onion and both black and white sesame seeds. Top with a few nori strips (if using).

Sea Vegetables

Consider seaweed. Nonadventurous diners who encounter a washed-up piece of it on the beach think of it as garbage, or perhaps more generously, as a snack for a gullible gull who hopes there will be a mussel attached. When we tramp across the same vegetation however, we are often reminded of our own dinners, and grow hungry at the thought.

Sushi eaters are at least a little more familiar with one kind of seaweed—nori—that is used as a binder for fish and rice. Seaweed or sea vegetables, as they are more stylishly referred to, are an absolute taste treat and, when combined as a salad, a veritable cocktail of vitamins, including the elusive B_{12}. Grown in oceans all over world, sea vegetables have an incredible complement of protein, minerals, and trace minerals; in fact, when raw and unwashed, a piece of seaweed will retain every single mineral held by the ocean, the structure of which is comparable to both human blood and amniotic fluid. Sea vegetables, which are macroalgaes, have properties that help the body keep cholesterol down and fight bacteria that has become resistant to penicillin. And the way it makes your hair thick and shiny is an added benefit.

Even if you've never been diving or snorkeling, thanks to *National Geographic*, The Discovery Channel, and *Spongebob Squarepants*, almost everyone can conjure up images of fronds that look like Matisse drawings, waving in the currents. Their colors range from yellow to green to purple, depending on the depth of the water in which they grow and how much light gets through to initiate photosynthesis. Most of our sea vegetables, including arame, wakame, and hijiki, are dried and then reconstituted; some, such as agar-agar, kelp, and nori, are ground, or shredded and, in the case of nori, pressed into sheets. And sometimes you don't even know the seaweed is there—Irish moss, for example, is harvested for its carrageenan, a thickening agent for soy-based faux-dairy foods and even shampoo.

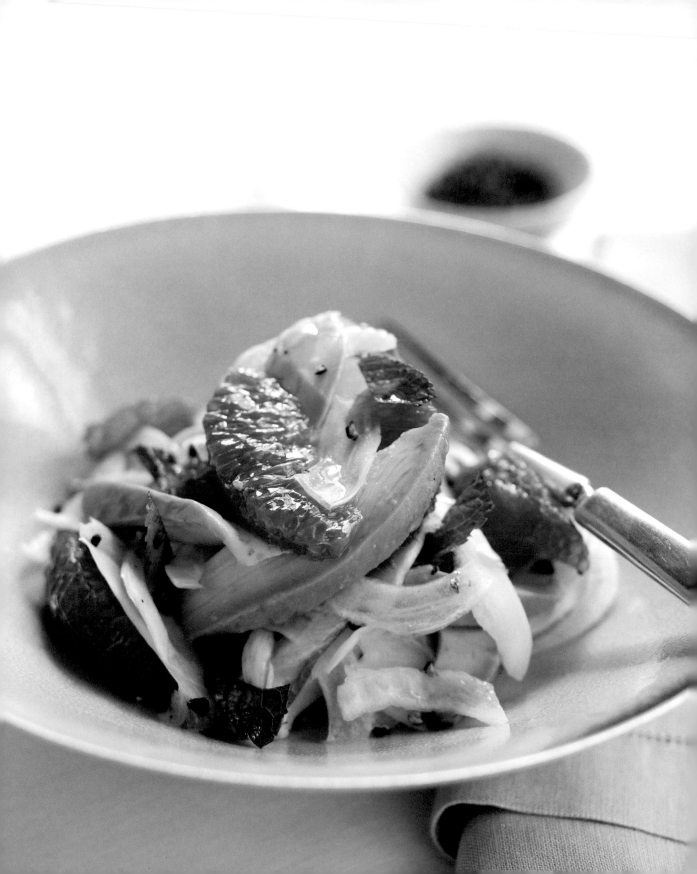

Red Grapefruit, Avocado, and Fennel Salad

SERVES 4

This recipe works equally well with oranges in place of the grapefruits. Blood oranges, if you can find them, are especially pretty. Macadamia oil is really nice in this salad, but feel free to use any other cold-pressed nut oil or high-quality extra-virgin olive oil. Cilantro or basil substitute nicely for mint. The cracked coriander is not necessary, but we recommend it for extra flavor.

3 large ruby red grapefruits or 5 oranges

¼ cup macadamia oil

1 tablespoon lime juice

Coarse sea salt

2 ripe avocados, peeled, pitted, and sliced

1 large or 2 small fennel bulbs, sliced thinly

1 very small handful mint leaves, julienned

Freshly ground black pepper

1 teaspoon cracked coriander seeds (optional)

Fennel fronds for garnish

1   To section the grapefruits or oranges, cut the peel from the top and bottom and stand each upright on a cutting board. Cut down from top to bottom along the peel to remove it and expose the flesh. Cut along each side of the membranes to separate the segments, and place the segments in a large bowl, along with any juice that you can squeeze out of what remains (sometimes it helps to carefully cut the grapefruit directly over a bowl). Set aside a few tablespoons of the juice to mix with the oil.

2   In a small bowl, whisk the oil with the lime juice, a few tablespoons of the grapefruit juice, and a generous pinch of sea salt. Place the sliced avocado in a bowl and pour some of the dressing over it, tossing very gently to coat.

3   Add the fennel, the remaining dressing, and the mint to the grapefruit and toss well. Gently combine the avocado with the grapefruit and fennel and divide among serving plates. Season with salt and pepper to taste, sprinkle with cracked coriander, if using, and garnish with fennel fronds.

Our Favorite Filling Salad

SERVES 2

This recipe is actually more of a list of suggested ingredients and options. Any quantities listed are just approximations. Use different nuts, or sunflower seeds, or no nuts at all. Add sliced radishes, fennel, or tomato. Skip the currants and toss in some finely chopped apple. Add microgreens if you can get them.

For both variety and nutrition, it's nice to try different types and arrangements of greens. Mix lighter greens with darker, heavier (and more nutrient-packed) greens such as kale, chard, spinach. It's also beneficial, for both flavor and nutrients, to throw in some spicy greens such as dandelion or mustard greens.

These are *big* salads. Since chewing is so important in order to maximize nutrient absorption and aid in digestion, we usually either read or watch something on TV while we slowly chomp and chew, like a couple of horses. And if you are making it for yourself and are not so concerned with making it look really pretty, use kitchen scissors to chop the greens, sprouts, and herbs together directly into the bowl (instead of chopping all the herbs separately). It's much easier to eat this salad if all the ingredients are in smaller pieces.

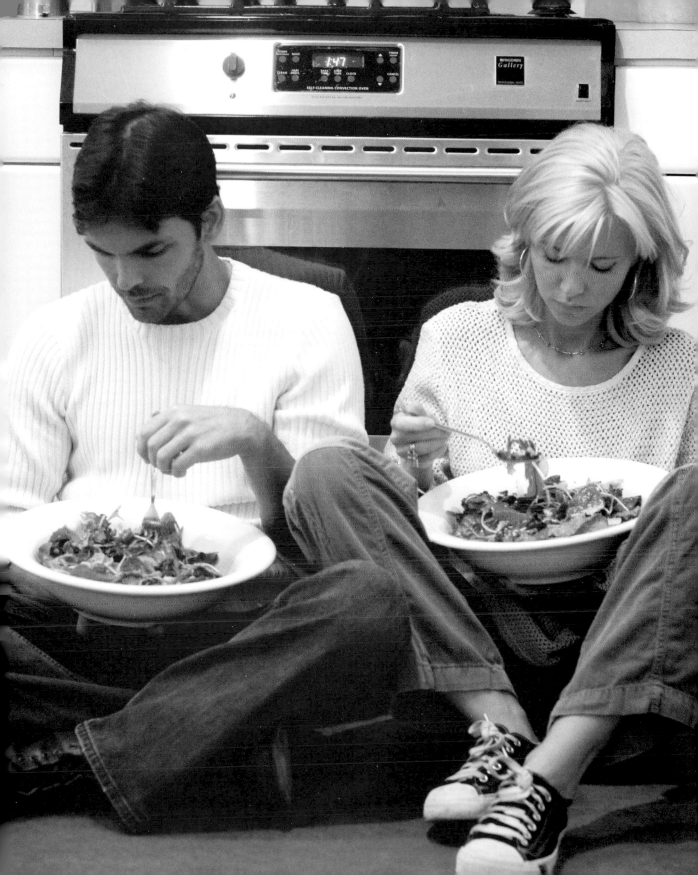

2 large bowls of mixed greens

2 handfuls sprouts, such as sunflower

¹/₂ bunch cilantro, chopped

¹/₂ bunch parsley, chopped

1 handful mint, chopped

1 handful basil leaves, chopped or torn

1 to 2 lemons, cut in half crosswise

2 to 3 limes, cut in half crosswise

¹/₃ cup macadamia nut oil

Coarse sea salt

1 to 2 ripe avocados, peeled, pitted, and chopped

1 large handful coarsely chopped dehydrated almonds or other nuts, or any flavored nuts
    from chapter 7, or a large handful crumbled Macadamia Cheese (see page 286)

1 handful dried currants

1 handful hemp seeds

1 large handful dulse, picked over to remove any shells and torn into pieces

In a very large bowl or two large serving bowls, add the greens, sprouts, and herbs.
Squeeze the citrus juices over the greens, drizzle with the oil, sprinkle with sea salt to
taste, and toss well. Add the avocado, nuts or macadamia cheese, currants, hemp seeds,
and dulse and toss gently to combine.

Chew on This

Our society may be speed-driven and oriented toward instant gratification, but that doesn't mean we have to swallow our food whole. We are not, after all, boa constrictors.

The digestive system works by delegation. Every organ has its job. The mouth is where food will encounter the first digestive enzymes. These enzymes immediately begin to break down carbs and sugars. So it stands to reason that the longer you chew, the more exposed your food becomes to deconstruction, and the more smoothly your stomach will be able to play its role. Those who bite and swallow without taking the time to thoroughly chew are being lazy bosses: they are handing out more work than they are doing themselves.

We're not telling you to turn into cows and masticate for hours on end. Just chew your food slowly and thoughtfully. If you treat your organs like treasured employees, they won't quit.

Microgreens

You may have noticed these incredible shrinking greens in your favorite fashionable restaurant, entwined with other ingredients as a salad or tangled on top of a piece of a fish as a garnish. Really, microgreens are a hipper version of that old health food staple, alfalfa sprouts, that have been given a not-so-extreme makeover. Instead of simply being sprouted to split open the protective shell, seeds such as alfalfa, sunflower, arugula, kale, broccoli, mustard, radish, or beet are grown into seedlings, then harvested (usually with scissors that won't harm the delicate stems) when they're about 10 days old. Voilà, miniature stalks and leaves that have yet to produce fruit and seeds of their own, so full of vibrant enzymes they practically quiver. Interestingly, along with nutrition, these Lilliputian plants deliver more of a punch to the palate than their grown-up siblings—the mustard is sharper, the arugula more peppery. On top of that, the fact that they are also so cute looking just adds to their appeal.

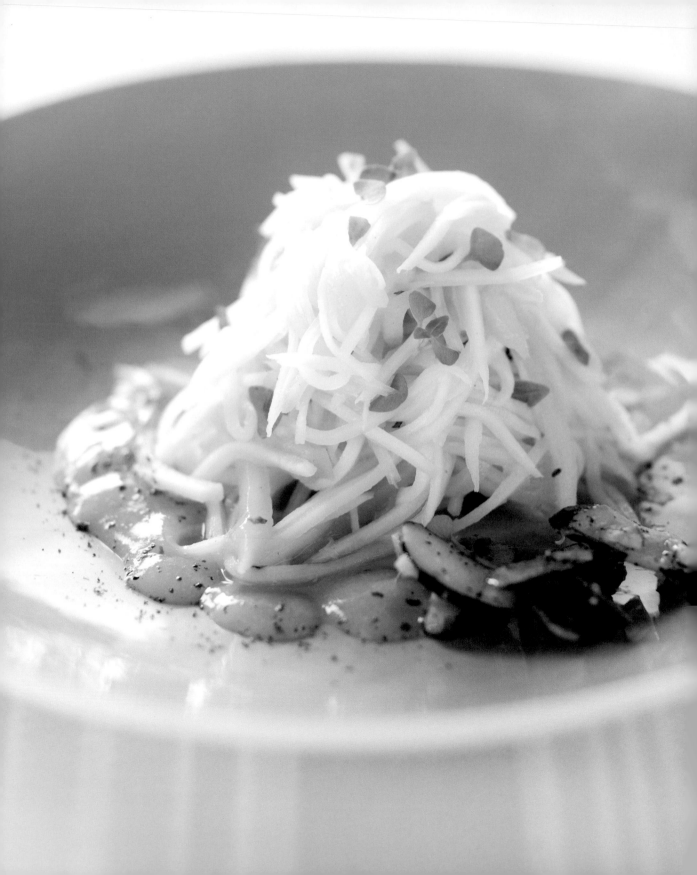

Double Mango and Thai Basil Salad

with red chile and star anise

SERVES 4

As Florida chef and cookbook author Allen Susser notes in *The Great Mango Book*, "In the world of mangos, there are two main kinds: green and ripe. Both are delicious, but they have very different uses. Green mangos refer to young fruit, usually pale green, without a hint of color; crisp, with a sour taste, although sometimes sweet and sour . . . ripe mangos are harvested when their skin grows yellow to orange and blushed." We like to use both in this recipe because of the textural contrasts—the apple-firmness of the green mango versus the banana-softness of the ripe one. You can find green mangos in Indian and Asian markets, as they are integral components in the cuisines of southeastern Asia.

If you don't have the time to dehydrate the spiced Brazil nuts that go with this, just dehydrate them as long as you can—the salad is still better with them, even if not fully dry and crunchy, than without. If you can't find Thai basil, any other variety will work fine, or try mint and/or cilantro.

1 cup Brazil nuts, soaked for 1 hour, thinly sliced

$^1/_3$ cup agave nectar or raw honey

1 teaspoon ground chili powder

Coarse sea salt

4 green mangos, peeled and thinly julienned

2 medium ripe mangos, peeled

1 small red chile

3 to 4 tablespoons coconut water or lime juice

Freshly ground star anise

1 small handful Thai basil leaves, thinly julienned

1 In a small bowl, mix the sliced Brazil nuts with the agave nectar, chili powder, and a generous pinch of salt, tossing to coat the nuts. Spread the nuts on a Teflex-lined dehydrator tray and dehydrate at 115°F for 24 to 48 hours. The longer they dehydrate, the crunchier they will be.

2 Place the green mangoes in a medium bowl and sprinkle with about 2 teaspoons of sea salt. Toss well and let stand for 30 minutes or more. The salt will soften the mangos.

3 In a blender, blend the flesh of one of the ripe mangoes with the red chile and enough coconut water to thin it to a smooth sauce consistency. Season with a pinch of salt and a pinch of star anise. Transfer the sauce to a squeeze bottle or separate container and set aside.

4 Cut the flesh of the second ripe mango into thin strips and add to the bowl of green mango, along with the basil, tossing to combine.

5 Paint each of the serving plates with the mango sauce, arrange a pile of the mango salad on each, sprinkle with the Brazil nuts, and garnish the plate with additional ground star anise.

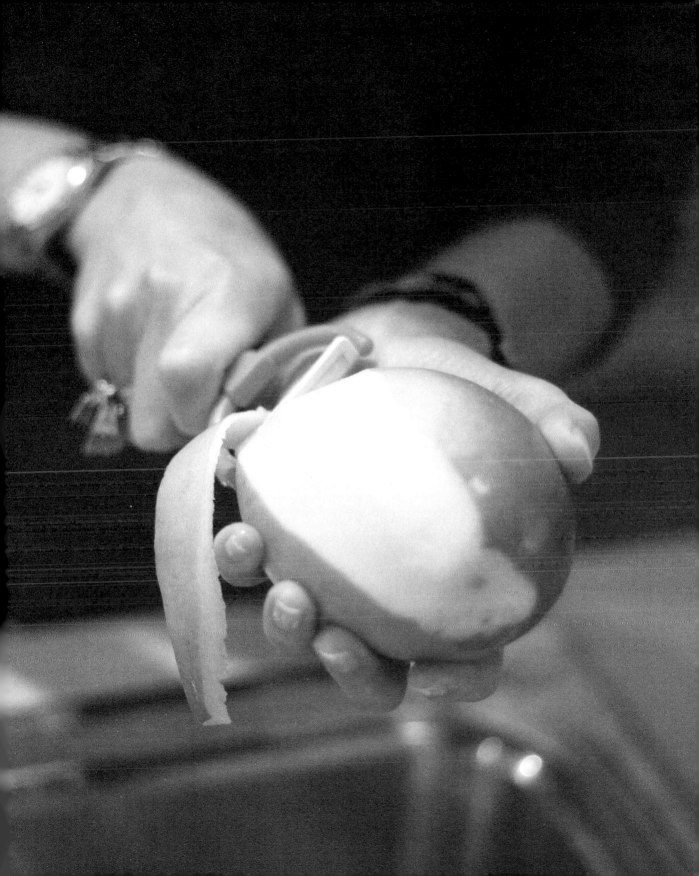

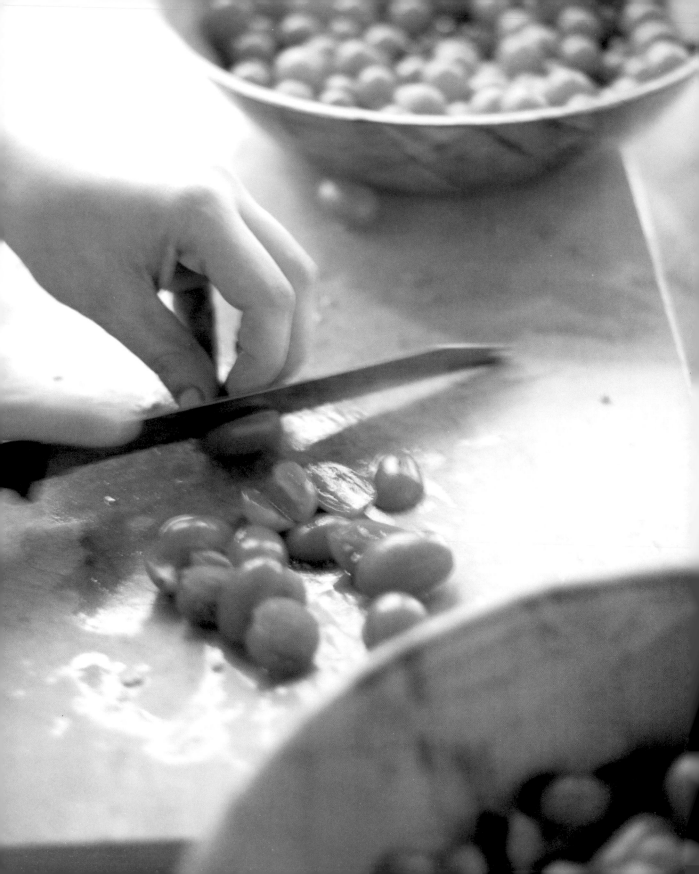

Warm Cherry Tomato and Sweet Corn Salad

SERVES 4

Along with the resurgence of oddly shaped, imperfectly delicious heirloom tomatoes, teeny tiny varieties have come back into vogue. Years ago we only had access to red cherry tomatoes, but now we are inundated with trendy teardrop, pear, poire-joli, currant, and grape tomatoes of varying sugars and acids, in hues of red, orange, yellow, and everything in between. For this recipe, any tomato that measures less than an inch in diameter is just fine—choose according to personal preference or what's available at the greenmarket. Although we recommend adding the crumbled macadamia feta, this is still a really good, refreshing salad without it.

3 ears fresh corn, husked

3 pints small cherry, teardrop, or grape tomatoes, sliced in half

4 tablespoons extra-virgin olive oil

1 tablespoon lemon juice

2 small or 1 large head butter lettuce, or other soft greens

3 tablespoons chopped fresh marjoram

1 cup crumbled Fluffy Macadamia Feta (page 288)

Coarse sea salt

Freshly ground black pepper

1   Cut the kernels from the corn cobs and place in a medium bowl with the tomatoes. Add 2 tablespoons olive oil and toss to coat. Spread the corn and tomatoes out on a Teflex-lined dehydrator tray and dehydrate at 115°F for about 1 hour.

2   In a large bowl, whisk together the lemon juice and remaining 2 tablespoons oil. Add the lettuce leaves and toss to coat well. Add the corn, tomatoes, marjoram, feta, and a generous sprinkling of sea salt and pepper and toss to combine. Divide among 4 serving plates.

Quinoa Tabouli

Traditionally tabouli is made with bulgur, or cracked wheat. As a substitution for bulgur, which can be difficult to digest, quinoa works very well and is extremely nutritious.

Sprouting is a technique often used in the raw food lifestyle. Soaking beans, grains, and seeds in water and then letting them sprout in the open air breaks down the complex proteins, carbohydrates, and cellular walls, allowing for easier digestion. To sprout quinoa, soak it overnight in water and then drain and rinse it in a fine mesh colander. Allow it to sit in the colander, draining over a bowl and covered with a clean towel, for at least 6 hours. Rinse once or twice, but don't rinse it right before you make the salad. It's best to have the quinoa on the drier side, so it will better absorb the lemon and olive oil flavors.

I have always loved Middle-Eastern foods. This salad makes a perfect and filling lunch served with Hummus (page 216) and Walnut Hemp Crackers (page 295). —MK

1 cup quinoa, soaked and sprouted (yields about 2 cups sprouted quinoa)
$1/4$ cup lemon juice
3 tablespoons olive oil
$1 1/2$ teaspoons sea salt
3 medium tomatoes, seeded and finely diced
2 green onions, white and 1 inch of green, very thinly sliced
2 bunches parsley, finely chopped
1 handful mint leaves, finely chopped

In a medium bowl, mix the quinoa with the lemon juice, olive oil, and sea salt. If you have time, let it sit for a little while to allow the quinoa to absorb the flavors. Add the remaining ingredients and mix to combine.

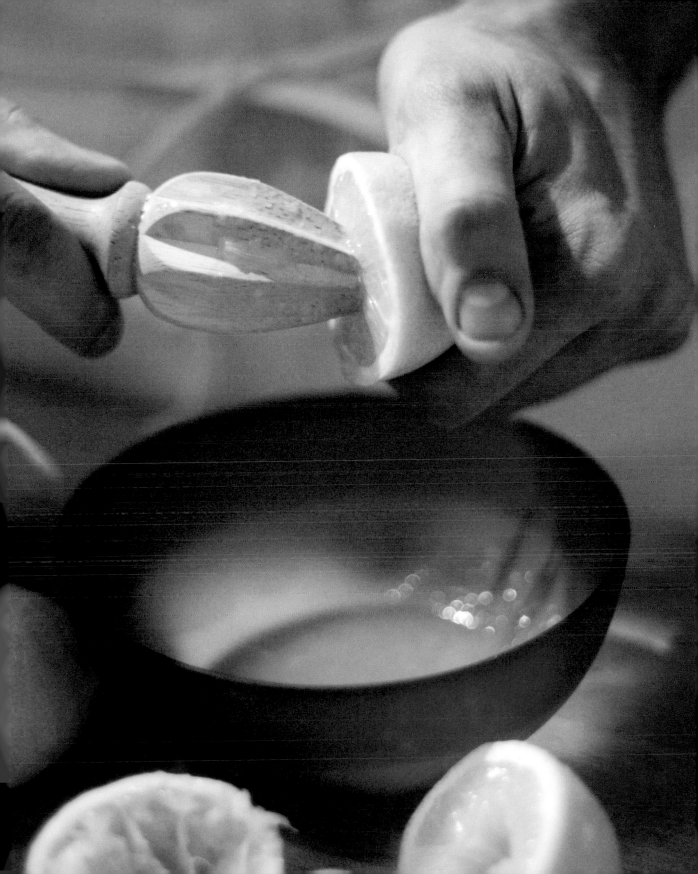

Quinoa and Grape Salad

SERVES 4 TO 6

According to our friend Renée Loux Underkoffler's *Living Cuisine* book, quinoa is not a grain but instead the seeds of an annual herb. It's actually easier to use than grains, as it's not heavy or sticky, and the protein is of very high quality. Quinoa is also a surprisingly good source for calcium, iron, B vitamins, and vitamin E.

This salad is a variation on a recipe from one of my favorite pre-raw cookbooks, *A Cook's Guide to Grains* by Jenny Muir.   —SM

1 cup quinoa, soaked and sprouted (page 120: yields about 2 cups sprouted quinoa)

$^{1}/_{4}$ cup lime juice

$^{1}/_{4}$ cup mirin

2 to 3 tablespoons macadamia nut oil or other nut or olive oil

$1^{1}/_{2}$ teaspoons sea salt

$1^{1}/_{2}$ cups halved or quartered grapes (red or green or a combination of both)

3 stalks celery, finely diced

1 large bunch cilantro, coarsely chopped

1 handful mint leaves, coarsely chopped

1 small handful basil leaves, coarsely chopped

1 green onion, white and 1 inch of green, very thinly sliced

1 large handful chopped, raw cashews (dehydrated, if preferred)

Freshly ground black pepper

In a medium bowl, mix the quinoa with the lime juice, mirin, oil, and sea salt. If you have time, let it sit for an hour or so to allow the quinoa to absorb the flavors. Add the remaining ingredients and mix to combine. If you are not serving this right away, you might want to leave the cashews out until serving, especially if using dehydrated cashews, as they will become soggy. Otherwise, this salad keeps very well for a day or two in the refrigerator. Taste and adjust seasoning, if necessary, before serving.

Protein

What about the question so often asked of vegetarians and vegans: "But where do you get your *protein*?" The World Health Organization reports that humans need 5 percent of daily calories to be protein. The USDA says it should be 6.5 percent. On average, fruits have 5 percent of their calories from protein; vegetables 20 to 50 percent, and sprouts, seeds, nuts, beans, and grains 10 to 25 percent. Getting enough protein eating only raw plant-based foods is not an issue. Plus, because the protein has not been damaged by heat, it is more effective for the body.

Greens are the ideal source of protein. Dark leafy greens in particular are very high in iron, calcium, folate, and beta-carotene. They are the best source of chlorophyll, a blood builder and natural healer. Their natural alkalinity balances the acids in our bodies (which on a pH scale actually prefer to be more alkaline), and promotes good health. When someone claims that we need animal protein for strength, you might want to point out the mighty apes. What do they eat? Mainly greens and bananas. No hamburgers or sushi. So it should not be inconceivable that we can thrive on plants.

As John Robbins asks in *Diet for a New America*, "Could it be that the whole issue of 'getting enough protein' is actually just a figment of our collective imaginations, with nothing behind it except for the propaganda of the meat, dairy and egg industries?" And he presents a very thorough explanation as to how and why that seems to be the case. Most of us are likely getting far more protein than we need. We have been conditioned to think that our bodies need *animal* protein, when in fact there is more than abundant research out there proving that we do not.

Amino Acids

Amino acids are the building blocks of proteins that you might remember studying in organic chemistry. When they combine into chains, they form the proteins that are necessary for cell, muscle, and tissue growth, repair, and restoration. Amino acids also serve as natural Prozac by helping form serotonin and dopamine, two neural hormones that govern our moods. The human body needs to acquire eight of these amino acids, which we call the "essential" ones, from outside sources; the other fourteen are built out of the first eight. But while all amino acids are good for the body, keep in mind that *how* they combine is the key. Their order in the chain is what differentiates animal proteins, whose amino acids are highly structured, from vegetable proteins, which contain free-form amino acids. Guess which one is easier to digest, contributes more to your overall energy level and increases both your beauty and well-being? That's right—plants, especially green leafy vegetables, are the best bricks for constructing your healthy foundation.

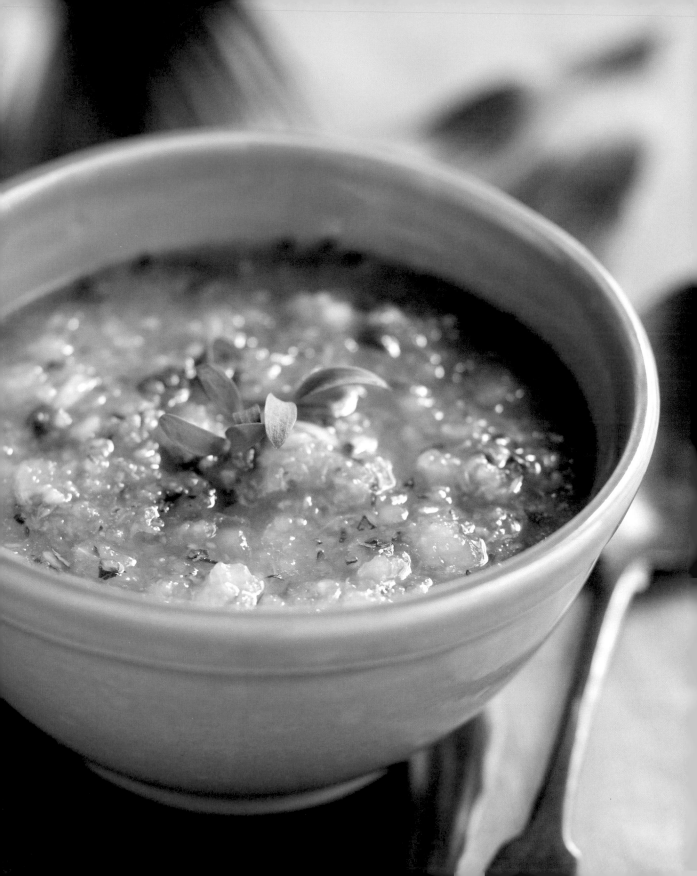

SOUPS AND STARTERS

All meals should begin with an impressive opening act. The goal is to seize the palate's attention, without overwhelming it, and raw foods are the perfect tools. Our first courses are colorful, small dishes, highlighting the use of fresh herbs, vegetables, and fruits in a variety of compositions. While these starters are modest in size (so that you or your guests will still have the room and desire for the next course), any of these dishes can be made into a light lunch or, in larger portions, a meal.

Some require a bit more time and planning than others—the Lobster Mushroom Tarts at the end of this chapter are probably not something you would throw together on a moment's notice, but they are worth the effort and gratifying if you enjoy the process, and of course, are satisfying to eat. Other dishes can be put together much faster, such as the soups. They are elegant, yet also easy to make and quick to serve—great for putting together ahead of time when you're expecting company. And because they are blended (and don't require too much chewing), they are a snap to digest, and good for the system if you're doing any sort of cleansing. Other dishes are great to share or to serve family style, such as the rolls, wraps, and sushi. And all of them can be varied according to your own imagination, using different herbs, spices, and other ingredients.

What really makes food preparation special is the creativity involved, the effort put into it, and the excitement of bringing something new and unexpected to the palate. For us, what we truly love about our restaurant and about taking the time to prepare this kind of food for friends and family is the knowledge that it is also so *good* for the people eating it.

Pineapple-Cucumber Gazpacho

with jalapeño, green onion, and cilantro

SERVES 4 TO 6

This gazpacho is best when chilled, so refrigerate it until you're ready to serve it. If you don't feel like breaking out your juicer to make fresh pineapple juice, or you don't have access to somewhere you can buy it fresh, just substitute an extra cup of fresh pineapple into the blender when pureeing—the juice simply gives the soup a smoother finish, but it will taste just as good either way. Because the sweetness of pineapples varies, the amount of jalapeño and salt may need to be adjusted to taste. We like to use Elysian Isle Avocado-Lime Oil in this recipe (see Sources, page 358).

I made this gazpacho the first summer we went raw, when I had been reading about how good and hydrating cucumbers are, and I wanted to combine them with something sweet and flavorful. I would be happy eating nothing but a big bucket of this soup over the course of a hot summer day. —SM

4 cups chopped peeled cucumber (from about 1 large English cucumber or a few Kirbys)

4 cups chopped pineapple (from 1 large or 2 small pineapples)

1 cup fresh pineapple juice

1 small jalapeño pepper, seeded and diced

1 green onion, white and 1 inch of green, chopped

1 tablespoon lime juice

2 teaspoons sea salt

1 handful cilantro leaves, plus a few extra for garnish

3 tablespoons avocado oil, macadamia oil, or cold pressed extra-virgin olive oil

1 handful finely chopped raw macadamia nuts

1 In a blender, add 3 cups each of the cucumber and pineapple, the pineapple juice, jalapeño, green onion, lime juice, and salt. Blend until smooth. Add the remaining 1 cup pineapple and 1 cup cucumber, the handful of cilantro, and 1$^1/_2$ tablespoons of the oil. Pulse the blender quickly a few times—the gazpacho should remain chunky. Taste for seasoning. If you have time, place the soup in the refrigerator to chill, or serve immediately.

2 Before serving, add the macadamia nuts to the gazpacho and stir to distribute them evenly. Divide among serving bowls and drizzle with the remaining 1$^1/_2$ tablespoons oil. Garnish with cilantro.

Watermelon Tomato Gazpacho

While seedless watermelons are much easier to handle, they are highly hybridized (the same goes for seedless grapes and citrus), which changes both texture and flavor. Hybrid plants are generally inferior to original wild plants, with less minerals and a lower life force. So for raw food purposes, they are an inferior product. Go for the seeds— after all, they're still fun to spit!

I'm sure this sounds totally cliché, but this soup is like summertime in a bowl. I love anything with watermelon, the single most refreshing fruit. Often, traditional gazpachos taste too Tabasco-y to me, but this one is spicy and sweet and fresh-tasting. Definitely serve it thoroughly chilled.   —SM

3 cups watermelon, seeded and pureed
   in a blender
1 cup seeded watermelon, diced small
1 cup seeded tomato, diced small
   (about 2 medium tomatoes)
1 cup peeled, seeded cucumber, diced
   small (from about $^1/_3$ English cucumber
   or 1 or 2 whole Kirbys)

$^1/_2$ cup red or green bell pepper, diced small
2 tablespoons lime juice
1 small handful cilantro leaves
1 teaspoon minced ginger
$^1/_2$ small jalapeño, seeded and minced
1 green onion, white and 1 inch of green,
   minced
1 teaspoon sea salt
Freshly ground black pepper

In a large glass bowl or container, combine the watermelon puree with the diced watermelon, tomato, cucumber, bell pepper, lime juice, cilantro, ginger, jalapeño, green onion, and salt. Stir to combine. Season with fresh black pepper and additional salt, if desired. Ladle into chilled soup bowls and serve, or refrigerate to chill and then serve.

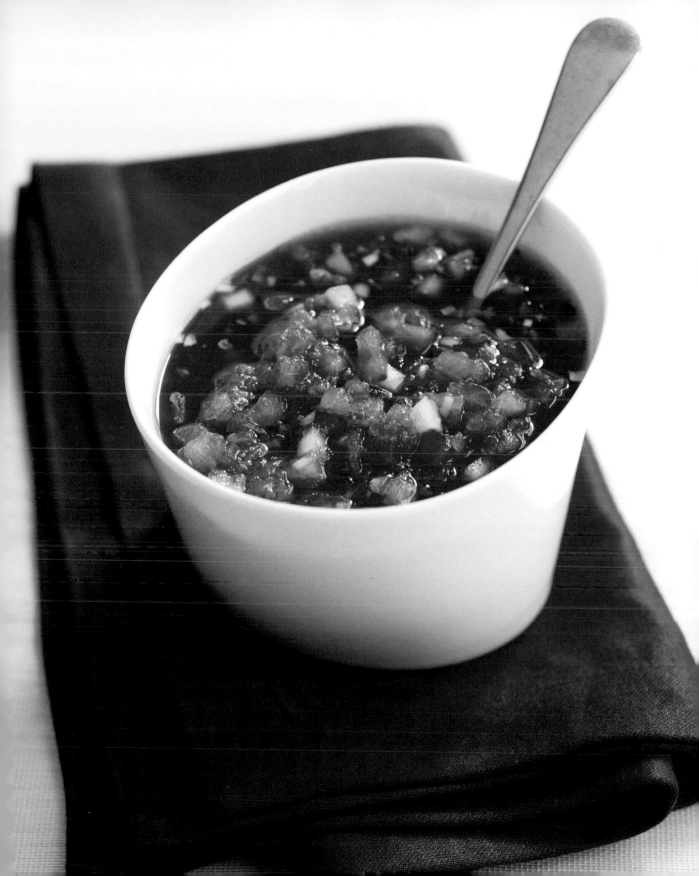

Raw Food and Wine: A Natural Match

Not all alcoholic libations are raw—some, like rum, are boiled in pot stills. But wine, which is fermented at low temperatures in oak barrels or stainless steel vats, is indeed an acceptable companion within the raw food guidelines. Even Western medicine readily acknowledges that the naturally occurring chemical compounds in wine, if taken in moderation, can help protect the heart from disease, and recent studies have pointed to wine being a satiating factor during meals. So from a lifestyle as well as a diet standpoint, *vino* is fine for the raw foodist.

That's the easy part. Pairing wines with composed raw food dishes is a little trickier. Clearly, the white-with-fish, red-with-meat credo doesn't work here.

If you are up to it, we suggest doing as aficionados do and go course by course, pairing each plate with a separate wine. Unless you're hosting the meal and need to pick the wines ahead of time, you can even wait until after you try the dish to order a vintage. This method allows you to first identify the strongest element, which may or may not be the main ingredient in the dish— herbs, spices, dressings, and sauces can easily dominate a recipe—and then complement that essence appropriately. After all it's not like your dish will get cold while you wait for your selection!

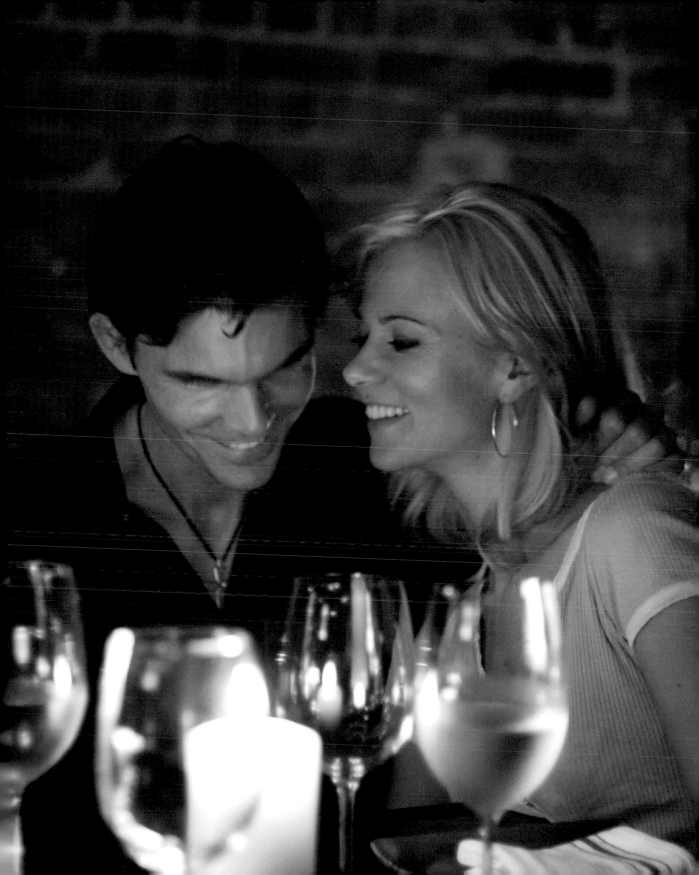

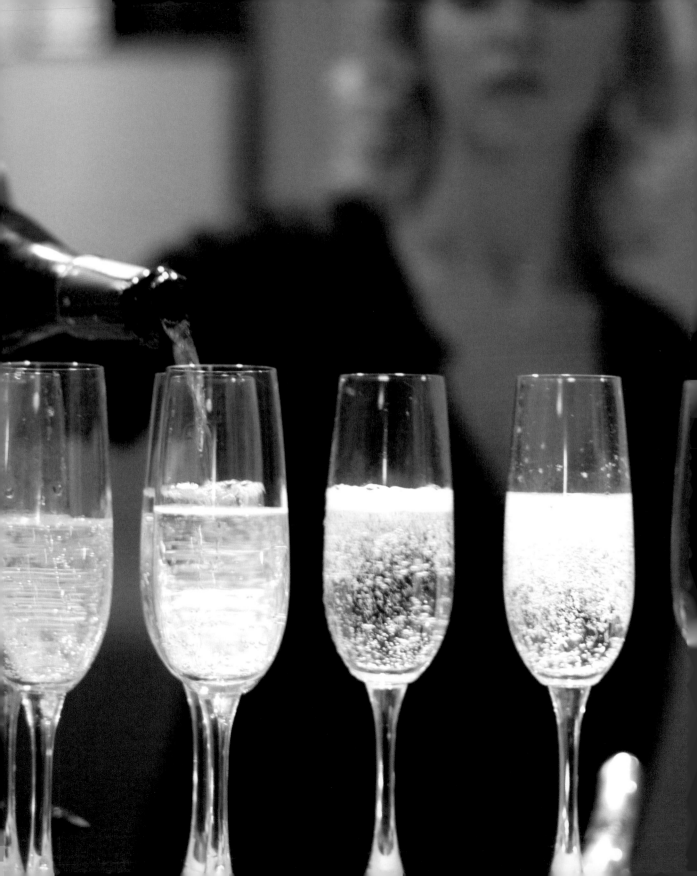

For instance, if you're starting off a meal with something fruit-based and acidic such as the Pineapple-Cucumber Gazpacho (page 128), consider countering with a varietal that offers some residual sugar, such as Viognier or Riesling. The rich and nutty Lobster Mushroom and Fava Bean Tart would go well with a red wine, such as an Austrailian Shiraz. A crisp champagne or sparkling wine is often a nice way to start off a meal, and complements the fresh and crisp Summer Rolls with Green Papaya nicely. A hearty main dish such as the Zucchini and Green Zebra Tomato Lasagne might call for a good, regional Italian red—say, an Amarone. Or for the Asian flavored Spicy Peanut Coconut Noodles with Ginger and Lime, try a dry sake (for more on sake, see Sexy Sake, page 325). We love dessert wines, and they pair nicely with the fresh fruit flavors of many raw desserts.

Of course we always recommend drinking organic wines and champagne when you can. More and more wineries in California and Australia are taking the technology out of the vineyards and returning to sustainable practices, resulting in an upswing of quality and quantity. And many Old World vintners are increasingly relying on biodynamics, in which seeds are planted and fruits harvested according to lunar and solar cycles (among many other cosmic forces). Both organically and biodynamically raised grapes make wine that is better for the earth, as well as our inner turf.

Creamy Carrot Ginger Soup with Lime

SERVES 2 TO 4

Serve this chilled in warm weather or gently warmed in cold months. The best way to heat a raw soup is to warm the bowl in which it will be served; if it's coming straight from the fridge, you can put it in a saucepan over *very* low heat, stirring it continuously for a few minutes, until it's warmed through. In this case, your finger is the best thermometer.

This soup is easy to make, has a beautiful rich color, and makes a soothing first course. The lime and ginger add freshness and spice. Although I prefer the added richness, the coconut is perfectly fine to omit if it is not readily available. —MK

3 cups carrot juice

1 small, ripe avocado

$1/3$ cup coconut meat

$1/4$ cup lime juice

2 tablespoons agave nectar

1 tablespoon minced ginger

$1/4$ teaspoon cayenne

$1/4$ teaspoon sea salt

2 tablespoons avocado-lime oil for garnish (optional, see Sources, page 362)

Few sprigs of cilantro for garnish (optional)

1 In a Vita-Mix or high-speed blender, puree all the ingredients until completely smooth. Taste for seasoning.

2 Divide among serving bowls. Garnish with a drizzle of avocado-lime oil and a few cilantro leaves in the middle and serve immediately, or gently warm the soup as directed above and then serve.

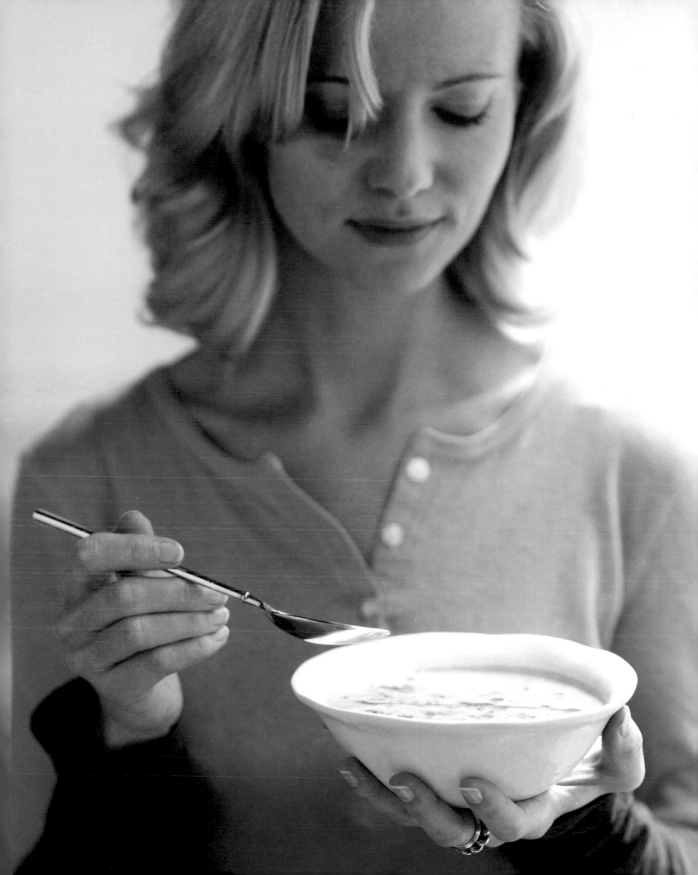

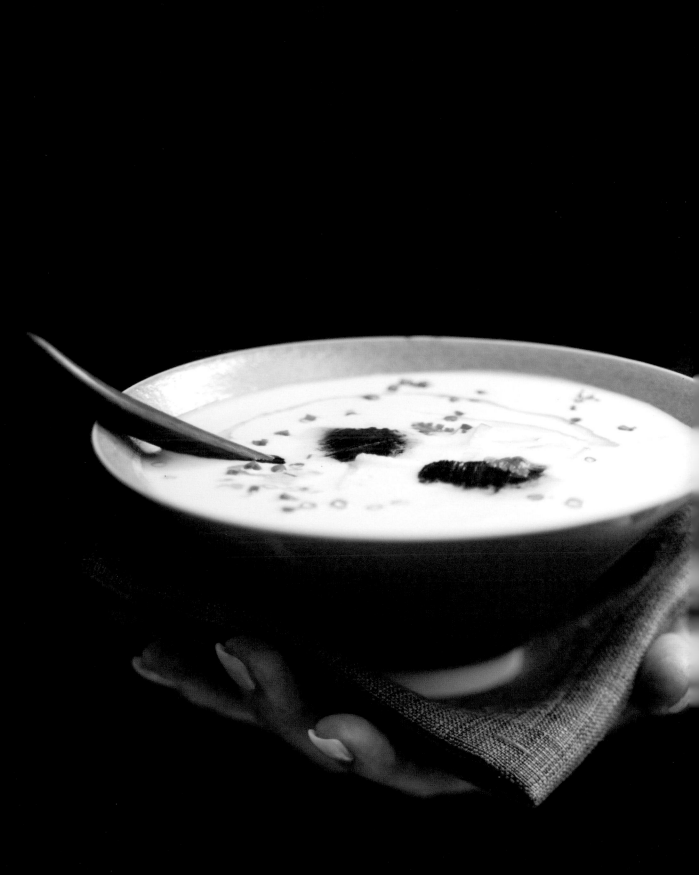

Celeriac and Green Apple Soup

with black truffle

SERVES 4

Celeriac, a member of the celery family, is an ugly, knobby root. It has a nice half-celery, half-parsley flavor, though, and is especially valuable as an ingredient in soups. Here, the woodsy, naturally salty freshness of the celeriac's essence complements the tartness of green apple and the earthiness of black truffles. In addition, celeriac is extremely low in calories, with no fat or cholesterol; immensely high in fiber; uniquely rich in flavor; and full of raw-recipe potential

As summery, light, and refreshing as the gazpachos
are, this soup is comforting, rich, and luxurious—perfect
for fall or winter. —MK

4 cups peeled, chopped celeriac
1 cup chopped green apple, plus $^{1}/_{2}$ cup very small dice for garnish
1 $^{1}/_{4}$ cups raw macadamia nuts, soaked for 1 hour or more
1 $^{1}/_{2}$ cups filtered water
2 tablespoons coconut butter
6 tablespoons extra-virgin olive oil
$^{1}/_{4}$ cup lemon juice
Sea salt
Freshly ground black pepper
$^{1}/_{4}$ cup minced chives
1 small fresh black truffle, shaved or julienned (optional, see Sources, page 366)
$^{1}/_{4}$ cup black truffle oil
Chervil leaves, or other herbs for garnish

1 In a Vita-Mix or high-speed blender, blend the celeriac and green apple until smooth. Pass through a fine strainer and discard the pulp. Pour the strained liquid back into the blender. Add the macadamia nuts, water, coconut butter, olive oil, and lemon juice and blend thoroughly. At the restaurant, if the soup still tastes a bit grainy from the macadamia nuts, we strain it again, but then add back a bit of the pulp and re-blend it to keep it creamy, yet smooth. This may not be necessary, just a matter of preference! Season the soup with salt and pepper to taste. If not serving right away, store it in the refrigerator in a covered container. Be sure to bring it back to room temperature before serving (reblending can help speed this process along as the movement increases the temperature) and taste again and adjust seasoning.

2 Divide the soup among 4 bowls, and garnish with the diced apple, chives, and black truffle (if using). Drizzle with truffle oil and top with chervil leaves.

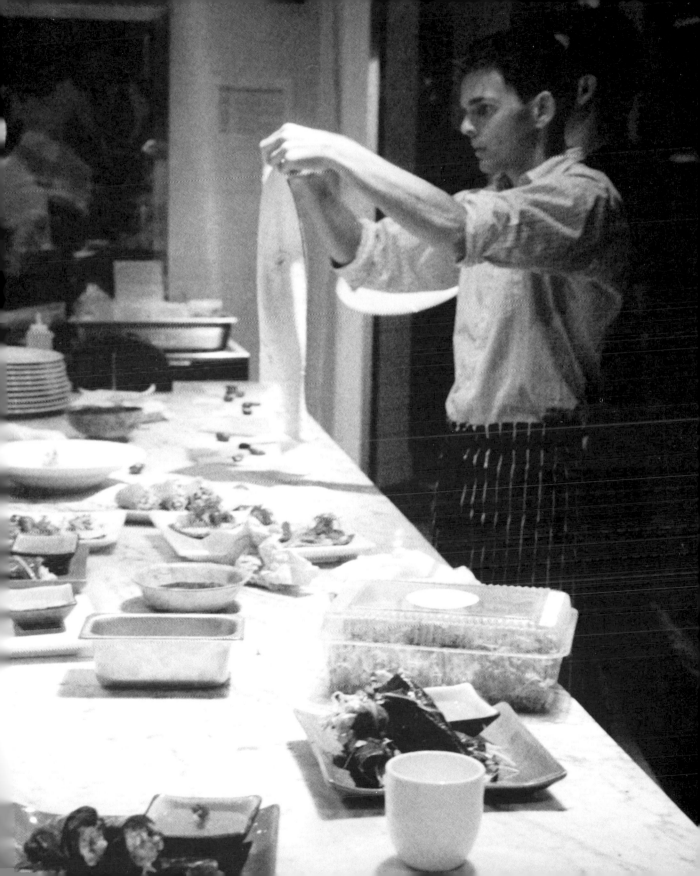

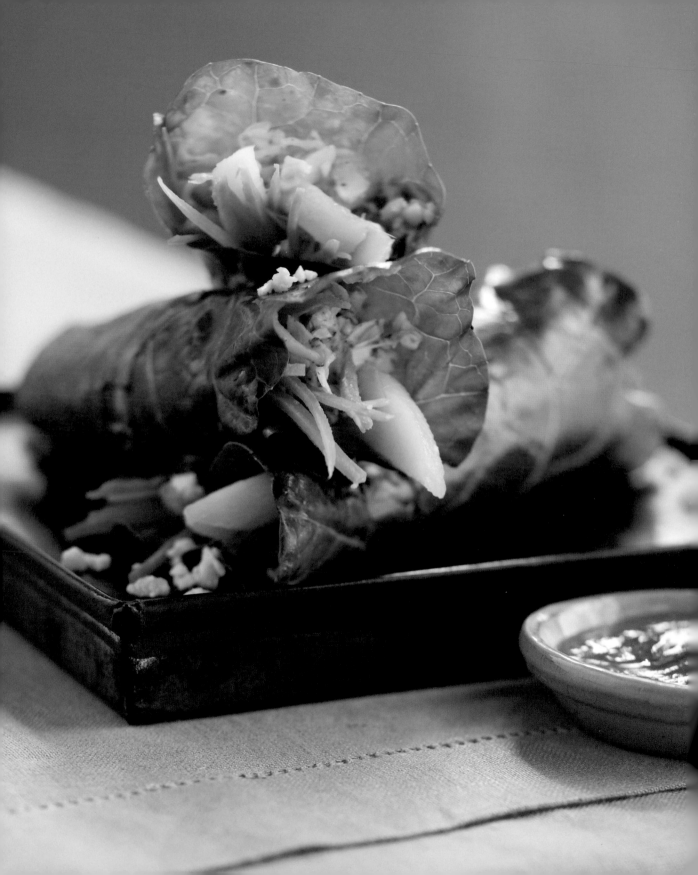

Spicy Thai Vegetable Wraps

with tamarind dipping sauce

Tamarind pulp can be found as cellophane-wrapped, sun-dried bricks in Asian, Latin, and Indian markets. Tamarind pulp is the sticky interior of pods that grow on a variety of evergreen tree originally native to Africa. Tamarind, which is very intense in flavor, lends sweet-and-sour notes to dishes. Because the pulp usually contains seeds, you should always strain it before use. Pull off an amount appropriate to your needs and soak it in warm, purified water for about 15 minutes. Then strain the pulp and liquid through a fine-mesh colander into a bowl to catch the usable diluted pulp, leaving the seeds and fibers caught in the mesh. (Discard what's left in the strainer.)

This is by far the most popular first course at our restaurant. I have to admit that it was somewhat inspired by Roxanne Klein's Pad Thai, in which she uses a bit of tamarind together with a spicy almond sauce. I had never really worked with collard greens before, but they were the biggest leaves I could find at the store, and happily they are a very sturdy, perfect wrapper. We make these to order at the restaurant, although they are still seriously yummy as leftovers the following day. —SM

For the wraps:

$^1/_2$ cup chopped raw cashews (dehydrated, if preferred)

1 tablespoon sesame oil

$^1/_2$ teaspoon sea salt

$^1/_4$ cup maple syrup

$^1/_2$ cup lemon juice

2 tablespoons chopped ginger

1 tablespoon chopped red chile, seeds included

$1^1/_2$ tablespoons nama shoyu

1 cup raw almond butter

$^1/_2$ head savoy cabbage, shredded

6 very large collard green leaves

1 large carrot, cut into matchstick-size pieces

1 large ripe mango, cut lengthwise into strips, about $^1/_4$-inch thick

2 cups bean sprouts

1 handful cilantro leaves

1 handful torn basil leaves

$^1/_2$ handful mint leaves (torn or cut if leaves are large)

1 In a small bowl, mix the cashews, sesame oil, and salt and set aside.

2 In a Vita-Mix or high-speed blender, puree the maple syrup, lemon juice, ginger, red chile, and nama shoyu. Add the almond butter and blend at low speed to combine. Add water to thin if necessary, to get a thick, cake batter–like consistency.

3 In a medium bowl, add the shredded cabbage and the almond butter mixture and toss well to combine (this is easiest if you use your hands).

4 Cut out the center rib of each collard green leaf, dividing the leaf in half. Place 1 half leaf on a cutting board with the underside facing up. Arrange a few tablespoons of the cabbage mixture evenly across the bottom third of the leaf, leaving about $1^1/_2$ inches clear at the bottom. Sprinkle some of the chopped cashews over the cabbage. Lay a few sticks of carrot, a few strips of mango, and a few sprouts on top. Add a few leaves each of cilantro, basil, and mint. Fold the bottom of the collard leaf up and over the filling, keeping it tight, and tuck the leaf under the ingredients and roll forward. Place the roll seam side down on a serving dish. Repeat with remaining collard leaves and ingredients. Serve with the tamarind dipping sauce.

For the tamarind dipping sauce:

1 cup soaked and strained tamarind pulp (see Sources, page 362)
3 tablespoons maple syrup
1 tablespoon nama shoyu
1 tablespoon extra-virgin olive oil
Pinch of sea salt

Place the tamarind pulp, maple syrup, nama shoyu, and olive oil in a blender and puree until smooth. Taste for seasoning and add a pinch of salt if necessary. Place in a separate bowl and set aside. This sauce may be made ahead and refrigerated for up to 2 days. It can also be frozen if you have leftovers or want to make it in advance.

Tomato Tartare

with green mango relish and macadamia milk

SERVES 4

This dish has roots—literally—in Thai cuisine. Galangal, a root similar to but a bit milder than ginger, is used frequently in Thai food. If you can't find it fresh, ginger is a perfectly good substitute. Kaffir lime is another traditional Thai ingredient. Both galangal and kaffir lime leaves should be readily available at any Asian market; if you can't locate them by sight, be sure to ask for assistance, or you can order them online (see Sources, page 359).

To make kaffir lime powder, place kaffir lime leaves in a dehydrator overnight until completely dried, and then pulverize in batches in a spice grinder or coffee grinder. It will keep in a covered container for months, like any other spice, and is a nice garnish to have on hand.

> **This is my favorite dish on our summertime menu at the restaurant—it's light and refreshing and elegant, yet complex at the same time with all the different flavor components. Valentin, one of our chefs, came up with this dish.** —MK

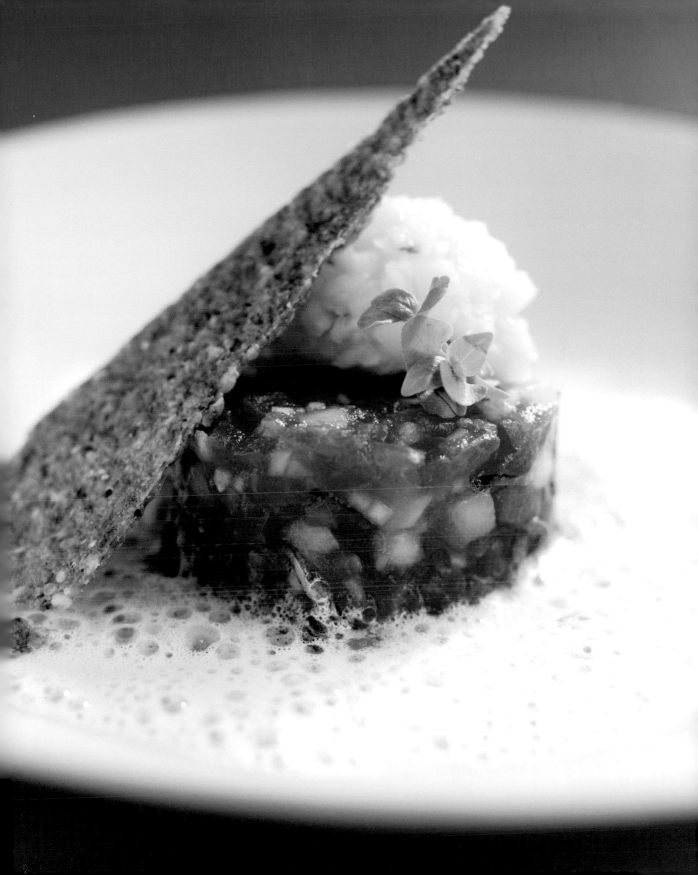

For the tomato tartare:

5 medium red tomatoes, preferably heirloom, seeded and cut into small dice
1 shallot, finely chopped
2 tablespoons finely diced green mango
$^1/_2$ cup of ripe mango, diced small
1 tablespoon minced galangal or ginger
1 small handful of Thai basil, julienned
2 tablespoons extra-virgin olive oil
Coarse sea salt
Freshly cracked black pepper

In a medium mixing bowl, combine the tomatoes with the shallot, green and ripe mango, galangal, basil, and olive oil. Season with coarse sea salt and freshly ground black pepper to taste.

For the green mango relish:

1 green mango, diced *very* small, or chopped fine in food processor
$^1/_4$ cup of ripe mango, diced small
1 tablespoon of Thai basil, julienned
$^1/_2$ teaspoon sea salt
Pinch of cayenne
Pinch of sea salt

In a small bowl, mix all the ingredients. Set aside.

For the macadamia milk:

1 cup macadamia nuts, soaked one hour or more
4 cups filtered water
2 large dates, pitted, or 2 tablespoons agave nectar or other sweetener
2 tablespoons lemon juice
Pinch of cayenne
Sea salt

In a Vita-Mix or high-speed blender, blend the macadamia nuts, water, and dates at high speed for at least 2 minutes. Strain the milk through multiple layers of cheesecloth to get rid of any grittiness, and season with lemon juice, cayenne, and salt to taste. Transfer to a covered container and chill in the refrigerator until ready to use.

For the assembly:

Walnut Hemp Crackers (page 295)
Microbasil, microgreens, or herbs for garnish
Extra-virgin olive oil for garnish
Kaffir lime powder (optional)

1 Place a 2 1/2 to 3-inch ring mold in the center of a coupe bowl or other shallow bowl and fill with the tomato tartare, packing it in with the back of a spoon. Carefully slide off the ring mold. Top the tartare with a small spoonful of green mango relish.

2 Foam the macadamia milk with a hand blender, or place it in a regular blender on medium-high speed to aerate it, or just put it in a sealed container and shake it up really well. Pour the foamed milk around the tomato, then garnish with the herbs and a cracker. Drizzle the milk with olive oil and sprinkle with the kaffir lime powder, if using.

Shiitake, Avocado, and Pickled Ginger Sushi Rolls

MAKES 6 TO 8 ROLLS

In this recipe, we call for *young* ginger, which is a paler, almost pinkish color, and milder in taste than mature gingerroot. Along with untoasted (and toasted) nori, you can find it at Asian markets, but the more commonly available ginger will work well, too. The beet juice used in pickling the ginger that goes into the rolls is optional, but we highly recommend it because it looks so pretty. And if you really want to cheat, you can just *buy* pickled ginger, if you can find any without preservatives.

If you can't find fresh shiitakes, you can substitute another wild mushroom or thinly sliced portobello, or even use dried shiitakes that have been rehydrated in purified water.

Wasabi is a very spicy variety of Japanese horseradish—fresh is best but it's hard to find and extremely expensive. You can buy powdered wasabi at most health food stores and Asian markets and mix with water according to the directions to make a paste.

Try other variations of sushi, using different vegetable fillings.

I like using jicama as a substitute for rice because it has a sweet quality to it that is similar to the seasoned sweetness of Japanese sushi rice. This is nice to serve if you are having guests. You can prepare all of the components ahead of time (except the avocado, which should always be sliced fresh) and then roll the sushi just before serving. We use biodegradable chopsticks at the restaurant that are made of corn and wheat—I love that. —SM

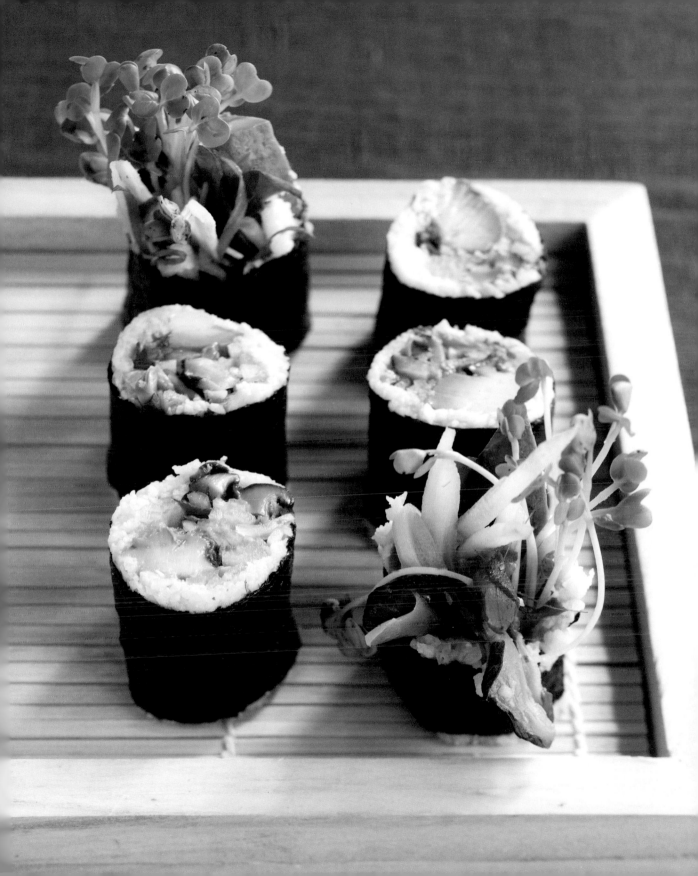

For the filling:

1 cup thinly sliced shiitake mushroom caps

$^1/_4$ cup nama shoyu plus $^1/_2$ cup for dipping

2 tablespoons extra-virgin olive oil

2 large young gingerroots, peeled and sliced very thin on a mandoline

2 tablespoons sea salt

1$^1/_2$ cups raw apple cider vinegar, or rice wine vinegar

$^3/_4$ cup agave nectar

$^1/_2$ cup beet juice* (optional)

1 In a small bowl, toss the shiitakes with $^1/_4$ cup of the nama shoyu and the olive oil. Allow to marinate for about 1 hour. Drain well and set aside.

2 Place the sliced ginger in a bowl and sprinkle generously with the salt. Let stand for about 5 minutes. Rinse well, drain, and squeeze out the water. Place about $^2/_3$ of the ginger in one bowl with 1 cup of the vinegar and $^1/_2$ cup of the agave nectar. Julienne the remaining ginger and place in another small bowl with the remaining $^1/_2$ cup vinegar and $^1/_4$ cup agave nectar. Add the beet juice (if using) to the bowl with the julienned ginger. Be sure the ginger is fully immersed in liquid—if not, simply add more vinegar and agave accordingly. Cover both bowls and refrigerate for at least 1 day and up to 3 days. Drain well before using.

If you don't want to get your juicer dirty for only one beet, grating it will work fine instead. Just add the grated beet to the vinegar, agave, and ginger. The color from the grated beet will seep out into the liquid and color the ginger almost as well as the juice.

For the rice:

6 cups chopped jicama (roughly 1-inch cubes)
$\frac{1}{2}$ cup pine nuts
1 tablespoon plus 2 teaspoons sea salt
$\frac{1}{4}$ cup brown rice wine vinegar
3 tablespoons agave nectar

1 Place the jicama and pine nuts in a food processor and pulse until chopped to the approximate size of rice grains. Press the jicama between clean kitchen towels or paper towels to remove all of the excess moisture.

2 In a large bowl, combine the rice with the salt, rice vinegar, and agave nectar and mix well. Gently spread the mixture onto dehydrator screens and dehydrate at 115° F for about 2 hours to remove additional moisture. It's a good idea to check the rice occasionally to make sure it is not getting too dry, and to toss it around a bit on the tray as the edges dry faster. If left too long in the dehydrator, it will start to turn pale brown, which is not really so bad, it just doesn't look as nice. If this happens, just add a bit more seasoning liquid, and keep in mind that the yield will be a bit less, and the texture not as soft. The rice will keep for up to 2 to 3 days in a covered container in the refrigerator. You should have about $4\frac{1}{2}$ cups.

For the assembly:

6 to 8 sheets untoasted nori
1 medium cucumber, peeled, seeded, and thinly julienned
2 ripe avocados, peeled, pitted, and sliced
1 small bunch sunflower sprouts or other long-stemmed sprouts
2 green onions, white and 1 inch of green, thinly sliced
1/2 cup wasabi
2 tablespoons black sesame seeds for garnish

1 Place a sheet of nori on a bamboo mat with the rougher side facing up; if you look closely, one side is usually smoother. Make sure the shorter side is closest to you (in art-school words, so that the nori sheet is portrait, not landscape). Place about 1/2 cup of rice on the nori and spread out evenly across the bottom third of the sheet, leaving 1 inch of space clear on the bottom. Lay some of the cucumber, avocados, shiitake filling, sprouts, and the pink julienned ginger across the rice. It's nice for presentation to let the leafy ends of the sprouts extend beyond the edges of the nori. Sprinkle with some of the green onion. If you like wasabi in your rolls, spread a small amount anywhere across the exposed nori before rolling (it is much easier to spread wasabi on the nori than to try to distribute it evenly with the rest of the filling, and it all ends up inside the roll either way).

2 Fold the bottom of the bamboo mat up and over the filling and roll the nori tightly. Wet the top edge of the nori with a little water to help seal it shut. Hold the roll in the mat for a few seconds to let it set and seal. Gently unwrap the mat, and using a very sharp knife, cut the roll into 6 pieces, wiping the knife clean with a wet towel between cuts. It helps to cut it in half first, and then cut each half into 3 evenly sized pieces.

3 Arrange the sushi on a plate and sprinkle with sesame seeds. Garnish with a small pile of the pickled ginger slices and a bit of wasabi.

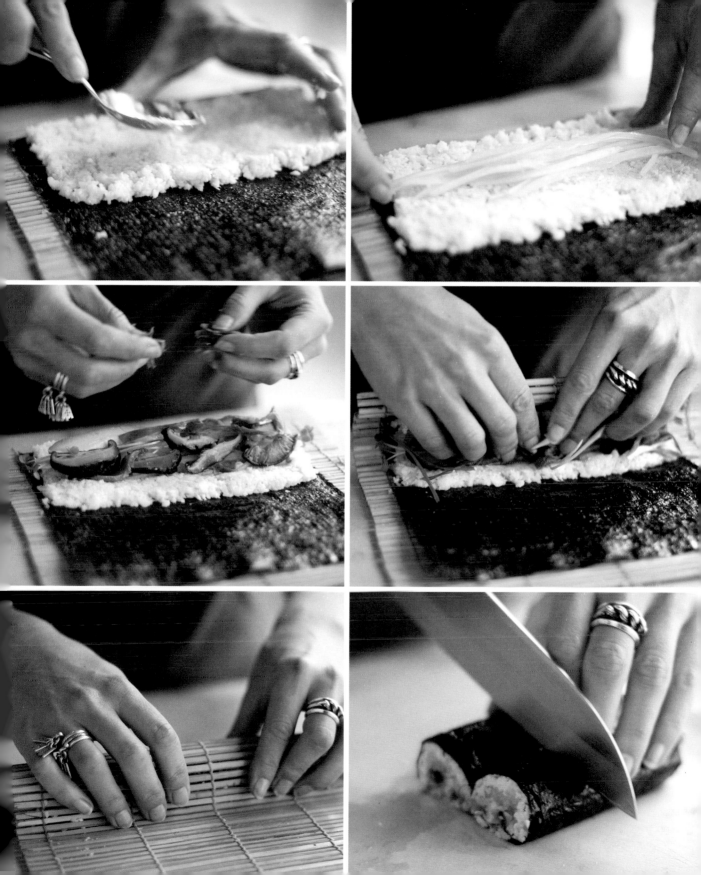

Summer Rolls with Green Papaya

SERVES 4 (MAKES 8 TO 12 ROLLS)

Our summer rolls are made with daikon radish sheets instead of rice paper, and they carry a fresh, satisfying crunch. At the restaurant, we use a very cool Japanese tool called a "sheeter" to make these wide sheets. They will hold any tubular vegetables lengthwise and cut very thin sheets with a long blade, but are a bit expensive and have many little, easy-to-lose pieces. Since most people probably don't have one of these kicking around in the back of the cupboard, you can jerry-rig sheets by overlapping slices of daikon or cucumber, cut thinly on a mandoline. And if you don't feel like making rolls, you can always toss all the ingredients and garnishes into a pretty salad. Dress it with a little dipping sauce and eat it with chopsticks or keep the dipping sauce on the side.

One of my first memories of eating Vietnamese food is of very fresh, crisp vegetables wrapped in soft rice paper and dipped in a tart, sweet plum sauce. Rice paper is very thin, and though cooked, would be such a small component of the dish that I wouldn't object to it as an acceptable wrapper for these rolls if you wish to use them. Either way, these are a great warm weather starter. —MK

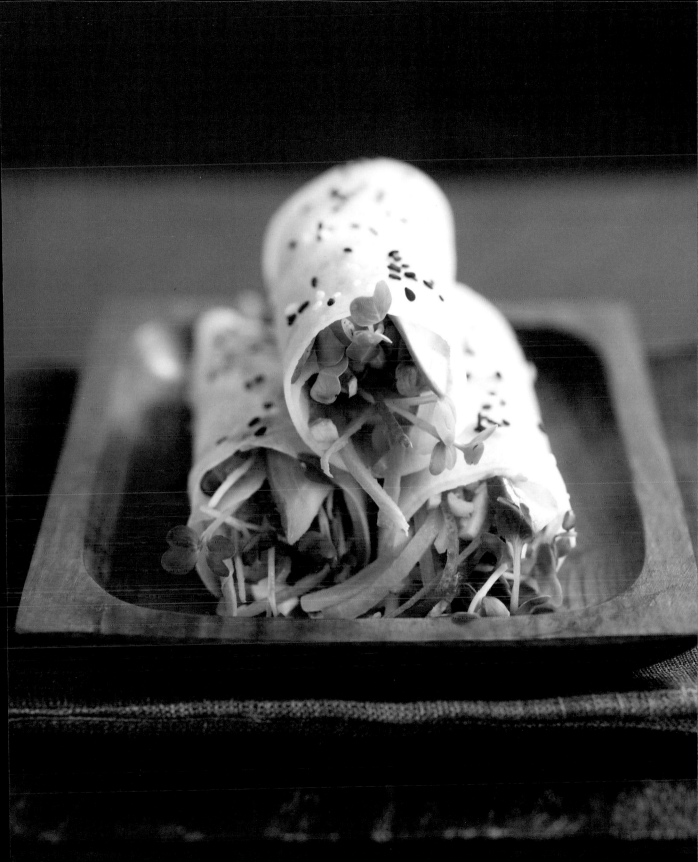

For the filling:

1 medium green papaya or green mango, peeled and julienned
1 cup julienned young coconut meat (see page 64)
1 large carrot, julienned
3 to 4 watermelon or other radishes, finely julienned
$\frac{1}{4}$ cup julienned ginger, plus 2 tablespoons finely minced ginger
$\frac{1}{4}$ cup nama shoyu
$\frac{1}{4}$ cup mirin
$\frac{1}{4}$ cup lime juice
2 tablespoons maple syrup
1 tablespoon sesame oil
1 long fresh red chile, seeded and minced
Sea salt
Freshly ground black pepper

1 Combine the green papaya, coconut meat, carrot, radishes, and ginger in a medium bowl and set aside.

2 In a small bowl, whisk together the nama shoyu, mirin, lime juice, maple syrup, sesame oil, and chile. Pour over the papaya mixture and toss gently to combine. Set aside to marinate about 30 minutes or longer. Drain before assembling the rolls.

For the red chili dipping sauce:

2 red bell peppers, seeded and chopped
2 fresh red chilies, chopped, with seeds to taste
$\frac{3}{4}$ cup young coconut meat
$\frac{1}{4}$ cup coconut water, or more as needed
Sea salt
Freshly ground black pepper

In a Vita-Mix or high-speed blender, blend the bell peppers and red chilies with the coconut meat until completely smooth. Add coconut water as needed to thin to a dipping sauce consistency and season with salt and pepper to taste. Transfer to a separate container and refrigerate until ready to use. Can be made up to 1 day ahead.

For the assembly:

1 large daikon radish, or 3 medium cucumbers, peeled
$^1/_2$ cup finely chopped almonds (dehydrated, if preferred)
1 tablespoon almond oil or other nut oil
Sea salt
1 ripe avocado, peeled, pitted, and sliced
1 handful Thai or other basil leaves
1 handful sunflower sprouts
2 tablespoons mixed black and white sesame seeds, or only black seeds

1 If using a Japanese sheeter, make daikon sheets and cut them into pieces about 6 inches long. If using a mandoline, cut the daikon or cucumber into very thin, lengthwise slices about 4 inches long. Pick out the widest slices to use.

2 In a small bowl, toss the almonds with the nut oil and salt to taste.

3 Lay out a sheet of daikon, or alternately lay down three overlapping slices of daikon or cucumber. Place a small handful of the filling mixture lengthwise on the slices. Sprinkle with almonds, top with avocado slices, basil leaves, and sprouts, extending the leafy ends beyond the wrapper by a little bit. Carefully roll tightly and repeat with remaining ingredients.

4 To serve, place the dipping sauce in a bowl or individual ramekins. Sprinkle the rolls with sesame seeds.

Lobster Mushroom and Fava Bean Tarts

with orange zest, cardamom, and chayote squash crust

MAKES ABOUT 6 TARTS

Lobster mushrooms are a big, meaty variety with coral-colored skins. You can use other firm, wild mushrooms instead of lobster mushrooms, such as chanterelles. We also like the unique flavor of huckleberries, which are not always easy to find. Substitute another berry, rehydrated dried cranberries or cherries, or try using the Balsamic-Fig Puree on page 194. If fava beans are not in season, you can easily replace them with asparagus, prepared in the same manner as for the Asparagus and Porcini Ravioli (page 193). Or you can skip them all together and add a few more mushrooms to the marinade. Be forewarned this recipe *does* take quite a bit of time and effort to prepare, so it's best suited for those who love the process as much as the end result (like us!).

One of our chefs, Valentin, used his superior skills as a technician to create this appetizer, which marries the earthy flavors of walnut, mushroom, and caramelized onion (made in our dehydrator) with the sexiness of orange zest and cardamom. It reminds me of my days preparing Moroccan-influenced food, which skillfully combines citrus, spice, and nutty flavors so well. —MK

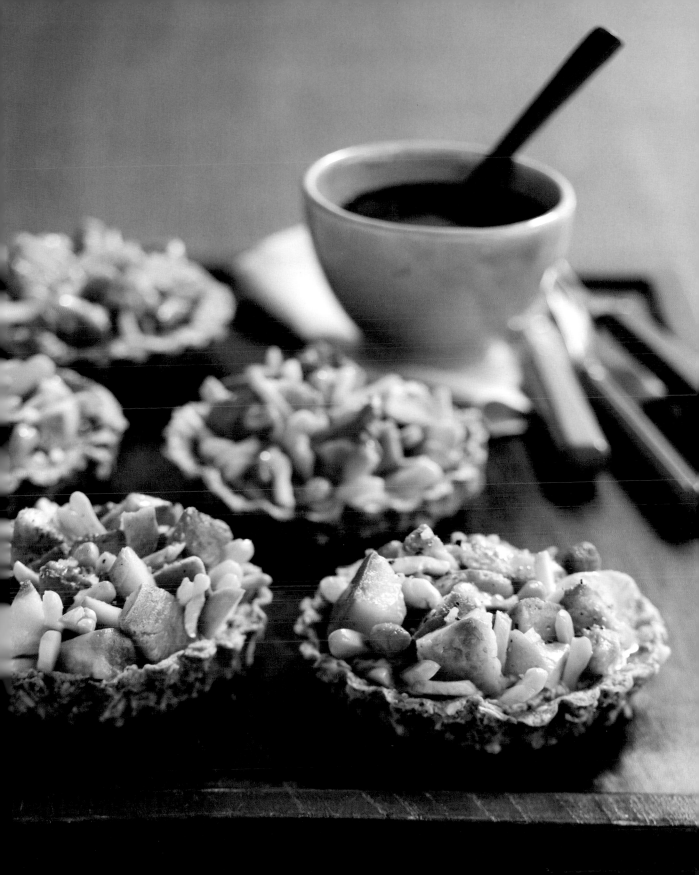

For the tart shells:

¹/₂ cup raw macadamia nuts
Pinch of sea salt
2 medium chayote squash, chopped (about 3 ¹/₂ cups)
³/₄ teaspoon ground cardamom
2 teaspoons grated orange zest
1 cup golden flax seeds, finely ground

1 Pulse the macadamia nuts in a food processor with the salt until the mixture resembles the consistency of couscous. Transfer the nuts to a separate bowl. Pulse the chayote in the food processor to medium-fine pieces about the size of rice grains. It's important not to process the squash too much or it will break down.

2 In a large bowl, combine the nuts and squash with the cardamom, orange zest, and about half of the ground flax. Mix well with a large spoon. Add more of the ground flax and continue mixing (you may want to use your hands at this point) until you get a dough.

3 Use 3¹/₂ to 4-inch diameter tart shells with removable bottoms. Fill each tart shell with a slightly heaping ¹/₄ cup of dough, or enough to line the shells about ¹/₄ inch thick. Use your fingers (wetting them with water helps) to push the dough into place to make a shell. Place on dehydrator trays and dehydrate at 115°F for about 3 hours or more. They should be dry enough to remove from the shells, which will help speed up the overall dehydrating time, but it's perfectly fine to leave them in a few hours longer. Carefully remove the crusts from the tart shells and place them back in the dehydrator and continue dehydrating until slightly crisp, 6 to 12 more hours.

For the filling:

3 small to medium onions
Juice of 1 lemon
$\frac{1}{4}$ cup nama shoyu
$\frac{1}{2}$ cup brown rice vinegar
$\frac{1}{4}$ cup agave nectar
3 cups walnuts, soaked for 2 hours or more
1 clove garlic, center germ removed
Sea salt
Freshly ground black pepper
1 small red chile pepper

1 Using a mandoline, slice the onions very thin. Marinate in enough warm water to just cover the onions, along with the lemon juice, for 30 minutes. Drain, then rinse twice in water (this helps to get rid of the raw oniony flavor). Drain again and place in a bowl.

2 In a small bowl, whisk together the nama shoyu, brown rice vinegar, and agave nectar. Add this mixture to the onions and let it marinate for 30 minutes. Drain the onions, but don't squeeze out too much of the liquid. Spread the onions on a Teflex-lined dehydrator tray and dehydrate at 115°F for about 24 hours, or until they are crisp and taste like caramelized onions.

3 Pulse the walnuts in a food processor with the garlic and a pinch of salt until they are tiny granules. In a blender, blend the onions with about $1\frac{1}{2}$ cups of water, the chile pepper, and a large pinch of sea salt. Add this liquid to the walnuts in the food processor and process for a mousse-like consistency. You may need to add more water. Adjust seasoning with salt and black pepper to taste.

For the topping:

¹/₂ **pound lobster mushrooms, or chanterelles**

Sea salt

2 small branches tarragon

2 sprigs fresh thyme

2 sprigs rosemary

1 bay leaf

1 garlic clove, center germ removed,
   smashed with the side of a kitchen knife

1 shallot, peeled and coarsely chopped

2 teaspoons black peppercorns

2 teaspoons coriander seeds

1 red bird chili pepper, coarsely chopped

1 cup filtered water

³/₄ **cup brown rice vinegar**

¹/₄ **cup agave nectar**

1 cup shelled and peeled fava beans

1 Clean the mushrooms, and cut them on a bias into bite-size pieces. Immerse them in cool water to rinse and get rid of any dirt. Drain the water and sprinkle the mushrooms with salt to taste.

2 Using a mortar and pestle, mash the tarragon, thyme, and rosemary a bit to release the juices. If you do not have a mortar and pestle, place the herbs in a bunch and squeeze and twist them with your hands (a bit like laundry), which also works well to help release their juices to more easily flavor the marinade. Make a bouquet garni by placing the herbs, the bay leaf, garlic, shallot, peppercorns, coriander seeds, and chili pepper in the center of a square of cheesecloth, pull the sides together, and tie it up like a little satchel. If you do not have cheesecloth, you can always use a coffee filter or place the herbs and other flavorings directly in the marinade, but it will take a bit more time to fish the mushrooms out after they have marinated.

3 Whisk together the water, brown rice vinegar, agave nectar, and a pinch of salt. Pour this over the mushrooms in a medium bowl and add the bouquet garni. Make sure there is enough liquid to fully cover the mushrooms. If not, add more vinegar, agave nectar, and water. Cover with plastic wrap and let sit for at least 1 hour.

4 Slice the fava beans in 2 or 3 pieces lengthwise and place in a small bowl. Sprinkle with a generous pinch of sea salt, toss, and allow to sit for 30 minutes or more.

5 Drain the mushrooms from the marinade and place in a bowl with the fava beans, tossing to combine.

For the huckleberry sauce:

$^1/_2$ **cup dried cherries or raisins**
2 cups huckleberries*
2 tablespoons red wine vinegar
Sea salt
Freshly ground black pepper to taste

1 Soak the cherries or raisins in water for 30 minutes or more to soften, reserving the soaking water.

2 Blend the berries, cherries, and red wine vinegar in a blender until smooth, adding a bit of the cherry soaking water as needed for a pourable sauce consistency. Season with salt and black pepper to taste. Transfer to a squeeze bottle or covered container and store in the refrigerator until ready to use. The sauce will keep for a few days if made ahead or if any is left over.

*You can substitute blackberries, but be sure to strain out the seeds after blending, or else blend for a sufficiently long time to break up the seeds, about 2 minutes. You can also use rehydrated dried cherries or cranberries with additional water, or use Balsamic-Fig Puree (page 194).

For the assembly:

$^1/_4$ **cup hazelnut oil or other nut oil to drizzle**
Sea salt
Freshly ground black pepper
Microherbs for garnish (optional)

1 Divide the filling between the tart shells and smooth it with the back of a spoon. Top with the mushrooms and fava beans. Drizzle each tart with about a teaspoon of nut oil, sprinkle with coarse sea salt and freshly ground black pepper to taste.

2 Place each tart on a plate, garnish with the huckleberry sauce and microherbs, if using.

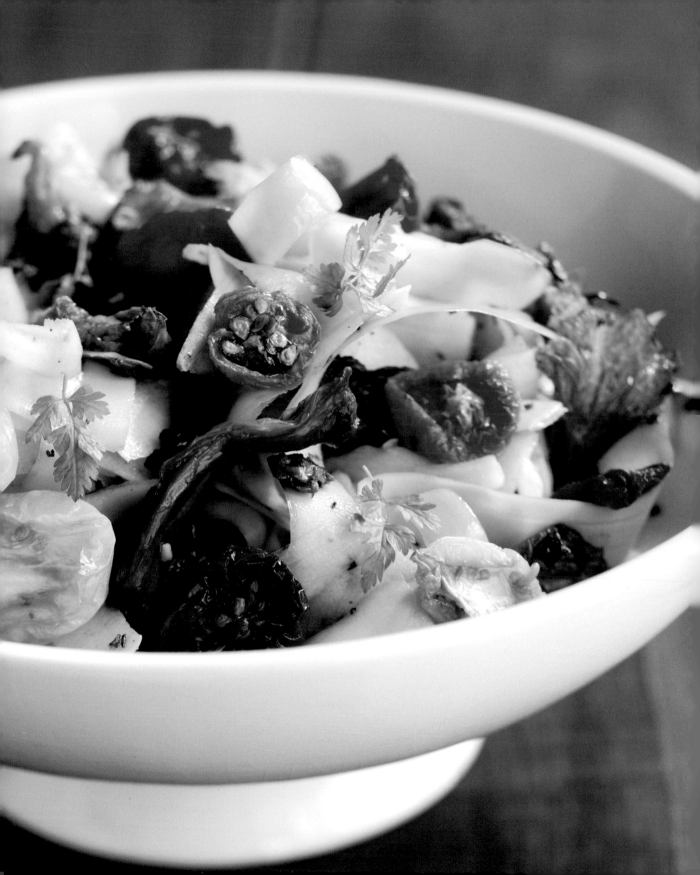

MAIN DISHES

Some raw foodists enjoy eating very simply, even consuming "mono-meals" such as a large bowl of cherries at one sitting, or a whole bunch of bananas or a few avocados at another. In some ways, this might ease our bodies' digestion, but it certainly doesn't make a raw food lifestyle seem particularly stimulating from a culinary point of view. Nor could we maintain a successful restaurant by serving plates of nothing more than our raw ingredients.

On our own, we might keep things straightforward by having a lightly dressed salad with avocado and hemp seeds, or a big bowl of summer tomatoes and radishes, simply garnished with sea salt and a good extra-virgin olive oil. We sometimes enjoy eating this way on a very warm day or when we feel our bodies would do well with something very simple.

When we share meals with our restaurant guests, friends, family, or business associates, a little more complexity is in order. We try to ensure that our main courses present a variety of textures, colors, and flavors, balance our affinity for sweet and sour, and satisfy our taste for salt and spice.

Given that the idea of raw food is unfamiliar to many, we also try to present our dishes in a style that is somewhat recognizable (lasagne, pizza), which helps people to visualize the food. We are not trying to mimic or create a substitute for the traditional versions (we don't aim to have our pizza taste like the kind made on a doughy white flour crust with gobs of melted mozzarella) and we like the freshness, complexity, flavor, and bright colors in ours better.

Don't feel compelled to follow each recipe as written. Numerous components from dishes throughout this book can also be enjoyed on their own as a snack, or combined to make a meal of tasting plates. For example, our cashew hummus, which we designed for our pizza, is excellent by itself, smoothed on a crispy cracker, served with a salad, or enjoyed as a dip for vegetables. Or make the guacamole from the tortilla recipe and enjoy it on its own with crisp, shaved jicama or romaine lettuce. Likewise the components of the lasagne (the tomato sauce, pesto, and ricotta) are all really good in a variety of other contexts. Use them together on a pizza crust or add herbs to the ricotta, which takes only minutes to make, and wrap it up in lettuce leaves. There are really endless ways to get creative with this food!

King Oyster Mushroom and Dried Cherry Tomato Fettuccini

with Cuban oregano

SERVES 4

This recipe calls for goldbar squash, a dark yellow, straightneck variety. Goldbar is an early season squash, so if you're making this dish later in the year, substitute regular summer squash. Avoid using a crookneck squash, as this will make your workload harder.

Cuban oregano is one of the herbs that we get at our local greenmarket. It has wider, plumper leaves with white edges—it kind of looks like oregano on steroids. If you can't find it, try growing it; Cuban oregano is an easy-care, vigorous plant that is virtually impossible to kill. It's okay to substitute common oregano, marjoram, or other herbs.

King oyster mushrooms are also called *saesongi* or *king eryngii* mushrooms, which are the names you might find them under in Asian markets. They have a long stem, thick cap, and dense, chewy texture. The Dlemal Mushroom Web site describes the lightly swayed shape of the king oyster as "a good and simple-hearted woman image." Not to argue semantics, but perhaps they should be called *queen* oyster mushrooms. Of course you can use any other mushroom, but the best replacement is matsutake or another sturdy field mushroom (not the common oyster mushroom, which is another species with a more delicate cap and tougher stem).

> " Zucchini would work just as well for this dish, or a mix of zucchini and goldbar would look pretty. " —MK

2 to 3 medium goldbar squash, ends trimmed

Sea salt

2 cups heirloom cherry tomatoes, stemmed and sliced in half

2 to 4 tablespoons extra-virgin olive oil

Freshly ground black pepper

2 cups king oyster mushrooms, stems removed and cut into bite-size pieces

2 teaspoons balsamic vinegar

2 teaspoons nama shoyu

2 to 3 whole stalks rosemary, plus 1 teaspoon minced

1 handful Cuban oregano, plus 2 teaspoons minced

1 shallot, minced

Fresh chervil or other herbs for garnish

1 Using a vegetable peeler or Japanese mandoline, cut the squash into wide, thin noodle-like ribbons, working around each squash until you get to the center seeds. Discard the center or save for another use. Place the squash in a colander, toss with about ¹/₂ teaspoon sea salt and let sit for at least 30 minutes to allow a bit of the liquid to drain out.

2 In a medium bowl, toss the cherry tomatoes with 1 to 2 tablespooons olive oil and season with salt and pepper. Place on the dehydrating screen cut-side down and dehydrate at 115°F for 6 to 8 hours.

3 In a medium bowl, toss the mushrooms with 1 to 2 tablespoons olive oil, the balsamic vinegar, and nama shoyu. Season with salt and pepper. Add the rosemary stalks, oregano, and shallot. Toss well, place on dehydrator sheets and dehydrate at 115°F for 3 to 4 hours, or until the mushrooms have softened and taste sautéed. Discard the rosemary sprigs and any larger oregano leaves.

4 To serve, toss the squash noodles with the mushrooms, tomatoes, minced rosemary, and minced oregano. Season with salt and pepper and garnish with chervil or other fresh herbs.

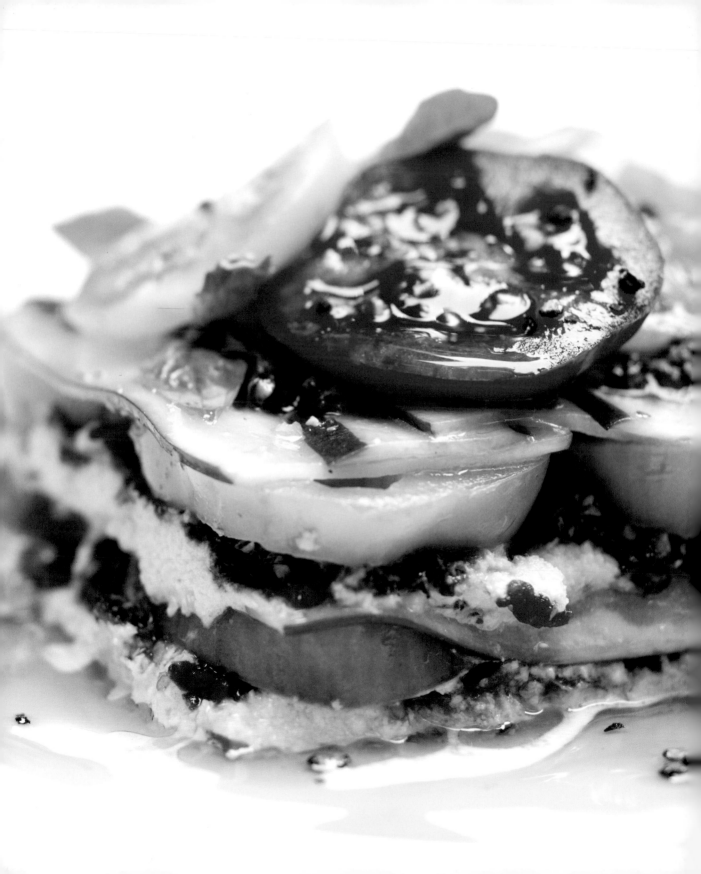

Zucchini and Green Zebra Tomato Lasagne

with basil-pistacio pesto, tomato sauce, and pignoli ricotta

SERVES 6

We like the vibrant color and tart flavor of green zebra tomatoes, an heirloom variety, for this dish. Of course you can use any tomatoes, preferably heirloom. Use the best quality sun-dried tomatoes you can find (but not the kind packed in olive oil, as this is most often not cold-pressed). The brighter ones make for a redder sauce, which will add good, Italian-flag contrast to the dish.

The first real raw food dish that we ever prepared was a rougher version of this. It has since become the best-selling dish on our restaurant menu and is a perfect introduction for anyone trying raw foods for the first time. The flavors and textures are all familiar, and the vibrant nature of the dish always leaves a strong impression. Many variations on this are possible. Feel free to add marinated wild mushrooms or substitute summer squash for zucchini. As in so many other dishes, the quality, seasonality, and freshness of the ingredients are the most important elements. —MK

For the pignoli ricotta:

2 cups raw pignoli (pine) nuts, soaked for 1 hour or more
2 tablespoons lemon juice
2 tablespoons nutritional yeast
1 teaspoon sea salt
6 tablespoons filtered water

Place the pignoli nuts, lemon juice, nutritional yeast, and salt in a food processor and pulse a few times, until thoroughly combined. Gradually add the water and process until the texture becomes fluffy, like ricotta.

For the tomato sauce:

2 cups sun-dried tomatoes, soaked for 2 hours or more
1 small to medium tomato, diced
$1/4$ small onion, chopped
2 tablespoons lemon juice
$1/4$ cup extra-virgin olive oil
1 tablespoon plus 1 teaspoon agave nectar
2 teaspoons sea salt
Pinch of hot pepper flakes

Squeeze and drain as much of the water out of the soaked sun-dried tomatoes as you can. Add the drained tomatoes to a Vita-Mix or high-speed blender with the remaining ingredients and blend until smooth.

For the basil-pistachio pesto:

2 cups packed basil leaves
$1/2$ cup pistachios
$1/4$ cup plus 2 tablespoons extra-virgin olive oil
1 teaspoon sea salt
Pinch of freshly ground black pepper

Place the pesto ingredients in a food processor and blend until well combined but still slightly chunky.

For the assembly:

3 medium zucchini, ends trimmed
2 tablespoons extra-virgin olive oil
1 tablespoon finely chopped fresh oregano
1 tablespoon fresh thyme
Pinch of sea salt
Pinch of freshly ground black pepper
3 medium green zebra tomatoes (or other heirloom variety), cut in half and then sliced
Whole basil leaves for garnish

1 Cut the zucchini crosswise in half, or into 3-inch lengths. Using a mandoline or vegetable peeler, cut the zucchini lengthwise into very thin slices. In a medium bowl, toss the zucchini slices with the olive oil, oregano, thyme, salt, and pepper.

2 Line the bottom of a 9 by 13-inch baking dish with a layer of zucchini slices, each one slightly overlapping another. Spread about $1/3$ of the tomato sauce over it and top with small dollops of "ricotta" and pesto, using about $1/3$ of each. Layer on about $1/3$ of the tomato slices. Add another layer of zucchini slices and repeat twice more with the tomato sauce, "ricotta," pesto, and tomato slices. Serve immediately, or cover with plastic and let sit at room temperature for a few hours. Garnish with basil leaves.

3 Alternately, to make individual servings, place about 3 zucchini slices, slightly overlapping, in the center of each serving plate, to make a square shape. Spread tomato sauce over the zucchini, top with small dollops of "ricotta" and pesto and a few small tomato slices. Repeat twice more. Garnish with basil leaves. Any leftover lasagne, whether made in a tray or individually, will taste great if kept in the refrigerator for at least a day or more, but it won't look as good (which doesn't matter if you're standing by yourself and eating it directly from the refrigerator, as we've been known to do at home).

Red Beet Ravioli

with cashew cheese filling, tarragon, and pistachios

SERVES 6 AS A STARTER OR 4 AS A MAIN COURSE

The colors in this dish are amazing: the bright blush of beets, the sunniness of yellow or orange pepper sauce, the summer-green herbs. When in season, experiment with candy stripe beets and try other herbs for the cashew filling. We use Sicilian pistachios that we buy at a Middle Eastern market (see Sources, page 361). They're a darker green and better-tasting than other types, especially when raw.

> Originally I tried to make red beet *gnocchi* using beet juice and ground up whole beets with other ingredients. They came out tasty, but our kitchen looked as if a gruesome crime had been committed. So I deconstructed the components a bit and came up with these much more manageable raviolis instead. —SM

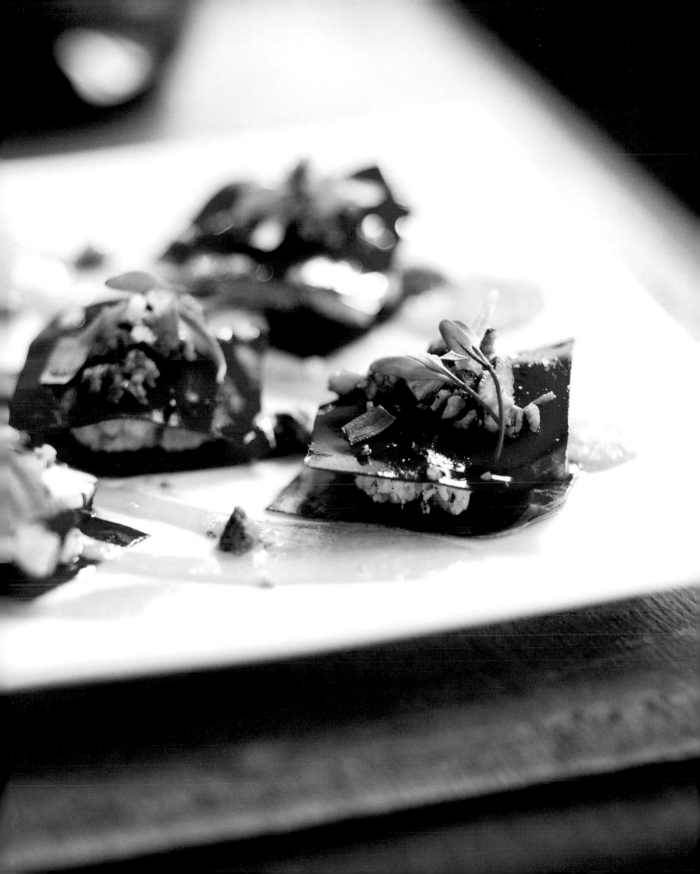

For the filling:

3 cups cashew nuts, soaked for 2 hours or more
$^1/_4$ cup lemon juice
1 tablespoon grated lemon zest
$^1/_4$ cup nutritional yeast
$1^1/_4$ to 2 teaspoons salt
2 green onions, white and 1 inch green, minced
3 tablespoons minced tarragon
2 tablespoons minced parsley

In a food processor, blend the nuts, lemon juice and zest, yeast, and salt until smooth. Transfer the filling to a medium bowl and fold in the onions, tarragon, and parsley. Taste for seasoning and add more salt or lemon juice, if needed. The filling should have the consistency of ricotta cheese. Store it covered in the refrigerator if not using right away; it tastes best if you bring it back to room temperature before assembling and serving.

For the pepper puree:

3 yellow or orange bell peppers, cored and cleaned
1 tablespoon lemon juice
1 green onion, white part only
$^1/_2$ teaspoon salt
1 tablespoon olive oil
$^1/_2$ cup pine nuts (plus 2 tablespoons, if needed), soaked 30 minutes to 1 hour
1 small pinch ground (or fresh) tumeric (optional, for added color)

In a Vita-Mix or high-speed blender, blend all the ingredients until smooth. If the sauce is too liquid, add an additional 1 to 2 tablespoons of soaked pine nuts. Place in a squeeze bottle or other covered container and refrigerate if not using right away.

For the assembly:

1 large bunch red beets (2 inches diameter or more)
2 to 3 tablespoons macadamia oil, other nut oil, or extra-virgin olive oil
1 to 2 tablespoons lemon juice
Coarse sea salt
1 handful chopped pistachios, preferably Sicilian
1 teaspoon pistachio, other nut oil, or extra-virgin olive oil
1 small handful fresh tarragon leaves, torn or left whole
Freshly ground black pepper
Microgreens for garnish (optional)

1 Using a mandoline, slice the beets very thin (about $1/16$ inch or less). Make stacks and cut into 2-inch squares. The size doesn't matter much, as long as they are all roughly the same. You should have at least fifty slices. In a medium bowl, add the beet slices, macadamia oil, lemon juice, and a generous pinch of sea salt. Toss to coat: there should be enough oil and lemon juice to coat all of the slices, but not so much that they are dripping in liquid.

2 Arrange half the beet slices flat on serving plates. Place a generous dollop of the filling on each slice. Sauce the plates with the pepper puree, using either a squeeze bottle or just spooning it over the beets and filling (this way some of the sauce will be inside each ravioli). Top each ravioli with a beet slice, pressing down gently.

3 In a small bowl, toss the chopped pistachios with the oil and a pinch of sea salt. Sprinkle each ravioli with the pistachios and top with the tarragon. Grind a bit of black pepper over the plates and garnish with microgreens, if desired. We use beet microgreens at the restaurant—they're pretty and delicate.

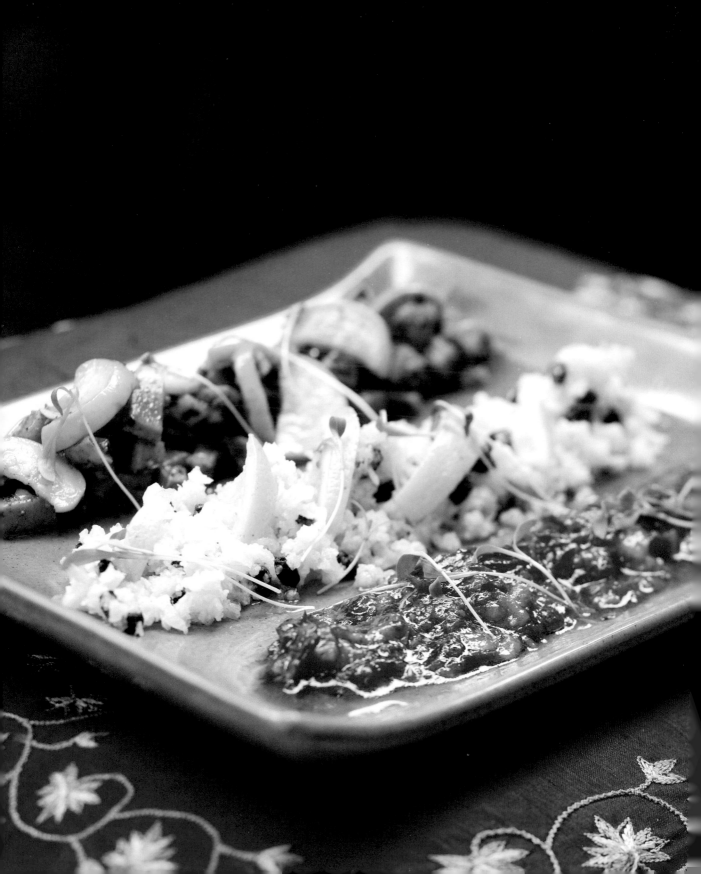

Pumpkin and Squash Couscous

with habanero harissa, currants, and almond oil

SERVES 4

The nice thing about this dish is that you can make any of the components separately and they stand on their own or complement other dishes. The spiced pumpkin seeds are optional, as is their flavoring—you can also season them with cayenne or other spices. However, preserved lemon powder is an unusual garnish and a nice change if you can find it. When you make this dish in the summer, instead of pumpkin use a mix of yellow summer squash and green zucchini or use baby pattypan squashes and baby zucchini, which we love.

The recipe calls for seasoning peppers—a variety popular in the Caribbean that is used more for its flavor than its heat. They are small and bright red, and can be spherical or long, and are sweet and very aromatic. If you can't find them, use additional habanero and red bell peppers.

Moroccan food has always fascinated me with its exotic, sensual flavors and its spirit, full of color and warmth. The jicama actually carries on the couscous tradition of being a light and fluffy vehicle for added, more intense flavors. We had not quite gotten this dish right when one of our sous-chefs, Louisa, came up with these vibrant accompaniments—a tangy, spicy habanero sauce and a floral squash-pumpkin garnish. —MK

For the habanero harissa:

4 cups roughly chopped seasoning peppers, seeds removed, or 3$^{1}/_{2}$ cups red bell pepper
   plus $^{1}/_{2}$ cup habanero
1 small roughly chopped habanero pepper, seeds removed
4 cups roughly chopped red bell pepper, seeds removed
4 cups roughly chopped yellow bell peppers, seeds removed
4 cups roughly chopped mixed red and yellow beefsteak tomatoes, seeds removed
$^{1}/_{2}$ cup agave nectar
1 shallot, crushed and roughly chopped
1 cup extra-virgin olive oil
Sea salt
Freshly ground black pepper

1 In a large bowl, toss all the chopped peppers, agave nectar, shallot, and $^{1}/_{2}$ cup of the olive oil. Season very lightly with salt and pepper. Transfer to shallow bowls or a glass baking dish and place on a shelf in the dehydrator. Dehydrate at 115°F for 8 hours or overnight, or until the peppers are softened and slightly dried. If you're available (or happen to wake up in the middle of the night), it's always a good idea to mix the peppers around every few hours.

2 Strain off any excess liquid. In a blender, grind the pepper mixture, adding the remaining $^{1}/_{2}$ cup olive oil while the blender is running to help it emulsify. Try to do this relatively quickly without overblending the sauce—it should have some texture to it. Season with additional salt and pepper, if necessary. Transfer to a separate container and set aside. If making ahead, cover and refrigerate up to 2 days.

For the pumpkin and squash mixture:

1 shallot, minced
1 tablespoon fresh thyme
1 tablespoon ground cumin
1 tablespoon ground coriander
1 teaspoon ground cinnamon
¹/₂ cup extra-virgin olive oil
¹/₄ cup almond milk (see page 57; optional for extra richness)
4 cups diced, peeled, and seeded pumpkin
4 cups goldbar squash or other yellow squash, cut into half-moons
Sea salt
Freshly ground black pepper
¹/₂ cup minced fresh parsley
¹/₂ cup minced fresh cilantro

1 In a small bowl, combine the shallot, thyme, cumin, coriander, cinnamon, olive oil, and almond milk, if using. Place the pumpkin and squash in two separate bowls. Divide the olive oil mixture between the two bowls evenly, and toss very well to combine. Season both with salt and pepper to taste.

2 Transfer the pumpkin, with the juices and oil from the bowl, to a Teflex-lined dehydrator tray and dehydrate at 115°F for about 6 hours, or until tender. Meanwhile, transfer the squash, with the juices and oil from the bowl, to a Teflex-lined dehydrator tray and dehydrate at 115°F for about 3 hours, or until tender.

3 When you are ready to serve, combine the squash and pumpkin in a mixing bowl with the minced parsley and cilantro, toss well, and check for seasoning.

For the couscous:

6 cups chopped jicama (roughly 1-inch cubes)
$^1/_2$ cup pine nuts
1 cup dried currants
$^1/_2$ cup almond oil
Coarse sea salt

1 Place the jicama in a food processor and pulse briefly a few times until chopped to the approximate size of couscous. Transfer to a fine-mesh colander and rinse for a few seconds under water to remove extra starchiness (this is not entirely necessary, but makes for lighter couscous). Press the jicama between clean lint-free kitchen towels or paper towels to remove excess moisture until the couscous is very dry and fluffy. Place in a bowl.

2 Process the pine nuts in a food processor until very finely chopped and add to the couscous with the currants, almond oil, and a generous seasoning of salt. This can be made ahead and stored covered in the refrigerator for a day or two. Be sure to bring it to room temperature before serving, and you may need to add more almond oil and salt, as the flavors always seem to mellow with time.

For the lemon spiced pumpkin seeds (optional):

1 cup raw pumpkin seeds, soaked for 2 hours or more
1 teaspoon sea salt
$1^1/_2$ teaspoons preserved lemon powder (see Sources, page 361)

In a small bowl, toss the pumpkin seeds with the salt and lemon powder. Transfer to a dehydrator tray and dehydrate at 115°F for 8 to 12 hours, or longer, until crisp.

For serving:

Microherbs, for garnish (optional)

Combine the squash with the couscous and serve with the habanero harissa, or, as we like to do at the restaurant, serve the components on each plate separately, to be combined as you eat them. Garnish with the spiced pumpkin seeds and microherbs, if desired.

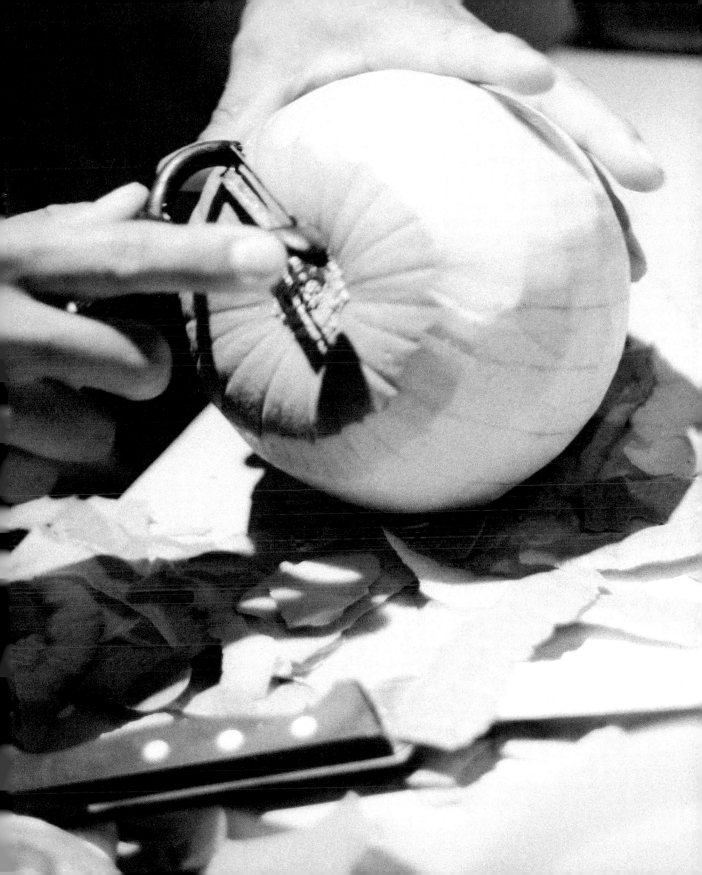

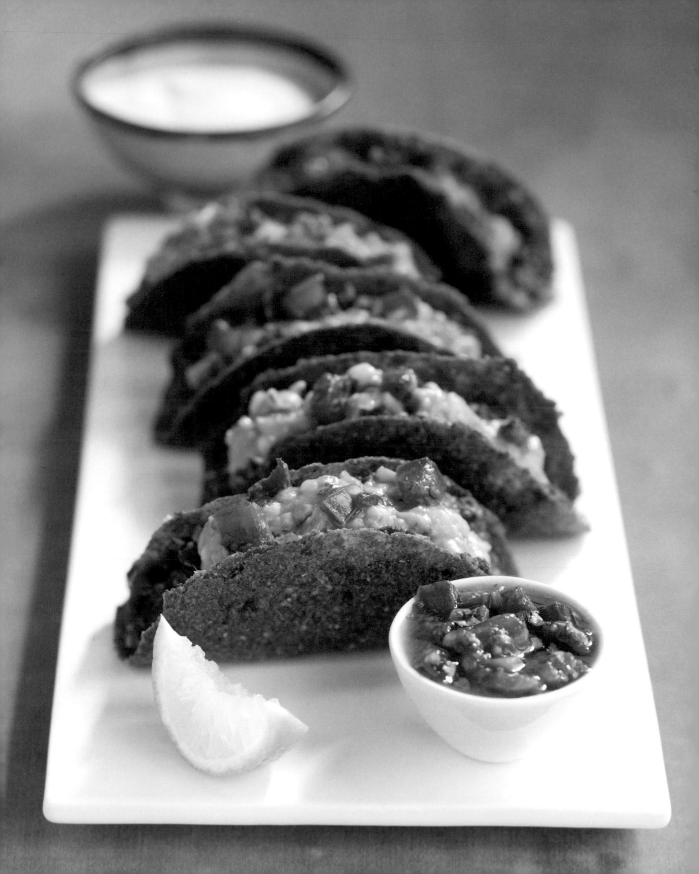

Soft Corn Tortillas

with spicy "beans," avocado-corn guacamole and tomato-lime salsa

Make this dish as spicy as you like. Don't cut too deep into the corncobs or you'll end up with those hard little pieces that get stuck in your teeth. When making the "beans," keep in mind that they will be tossed with a mild tomato sauce, so the spiciness will be mellowed out. If you want to make them ahead of time, keep all the components separate and assemble at the last minute, as the tortillas will get soggy if left to sit too long. The flaxseed can be ground in a coffee or spice grinder or Vita-Mix with dry blade (it will yield about 1 cup ground flaxseed).

We sometimes get large, skeptical men in the restaurant who may have been dragged in by a girlfriend or family member and who proudly insist 'I'm a meat and potatoes guy!' For them, I always recommend this particular dish. It's very filling and hearty. Then I smile graciously as the same guys later inevitably tell me something like, 'I thought I was going to have to go for a burger after this, but I'm really full!' I've had so many variations of this conversation, and it's always the tortillas that get the best response from the self-proclaimed 'carnivores.' —SM

For the corn tortillas:

3 cups fresh corn kernels, cut from
      2–3 ears, or thawed frozen corn
1¹/₂ cups chopped yellow or red bell pepper
³/₄ cup golden flaxseed, finely ground

1 tablespoon lime juice
1 tablespoon ground chili powder
1¹/₂ teaspoons sea salt
2 teaspoons ground cumin

1 In a food processor, chop the corn and bell pepper. Add the remaining ingredients and process until almost smooth.

2 Divide the dough onto two Teflex-lined dehydrator trays and spread to the edges using an offset spatula. Dehydrate at 115°F for 3 to 4 hours. Flip the Teflex sheets over onto the tray and carefully peel away the Teflex. Place back in the dehydrator for about 2 hours.

3 When the tortilla is completely dry on both sides but still pliable, remove it from the dehydrator and place on a flat surface. Use a round cutter or small plate about 4 inches in diameter and trace around it with a knife to cut round tortillas. You should have about 9 tortillas per 14-inch tray. Keep the scraps to add to a salad or just eat them plain as a snack.

For the spicy "beans":

1¹/₂ cups sunflower seeds, soaked for
      2 hours or more
1 cup sun-dried tomatoes, soaked for
      1 hour or more
1 tablespoon miso
2 teaspoons ground cumin
2 teaspoons ancho chili powder
2 teaspoons ground coriander

1 teaspoon cayenne pepper
2 tablespoons olive oil
1 tablespoon agave nectar
1 teaspoon sea salt
6 tablespoons filtered water
¹/₂ to 1 jalapeño, cored but with seeds, chopped
3 green onions, chopped
1 small handful fresh cilantro

1 In a food processor, grind the sunflower seeds, tomatoes, miso, cumin, chile powder, coriander, cayenne, olive oil, agave nectar, and sea salt until thoroughly combined. Add the water a few tablespoons at a time and process further for a wet dough-like consistency. Taste for seasoning. Add the jalapeño, green onions, and cilantro and pulse a few times to combine, but leave small bits of herbs.

2 Spoon the mixture onto 1 or 2 Teflex-lined dehydrator trays. You don't need to smooth it out; leave it chunky on the tray but flat enough to fit under another tray. Dehydrate at 115°F overnight, or about 10 hours. If possible, about halfway through, flip the "bean" mix over so the undersides can dry—this step is not totally necessary, as the mix will be combined with the wet tomato sauce anyhow. The mix should be dry on the outside and not too mushy, so it can be broken up into pieces.

For the tomato sauce:

2 cups sun-dried tomatoes, soaked for at least 1 hour
1 small tomato, chopped
¼ medium onion, chopped
2 tablespoons lemon juice
1 teaspoon sea salt
Pinch of hot pepper flakes

1 Place all the sauce ingredients in a food processor and grind well to a thick sauce consistency.

2 Place the "bean" mix in a medium bowl and break up any larger pieces. Add the tomato sauce and toss to combine well. It should be thick and somewhat spreadable. If not using right away, cover and store in the refrigerator for up to a few days, if necessary.

For the avocado-corn guacamole:

3 ripe avocados, pitted
1 cup fresh corn kernels, cut from 1 ear (or use thawed frozen corn or simply omit)
1 large handful cilantro leaves, finely chopped
2 tablespoons lime juice
½ jalapeño pepper, finely minced
1 teaspoon sea salt

In a medium bowl, mash the avocados well with a fork. Add the corn, cilantro, lime juice, jalapeño, and salt and stir well to combine. If not using immediately, cover the surface of the guacamole with plastic wrap and refrigerate. This will only keep well for about a day or so.

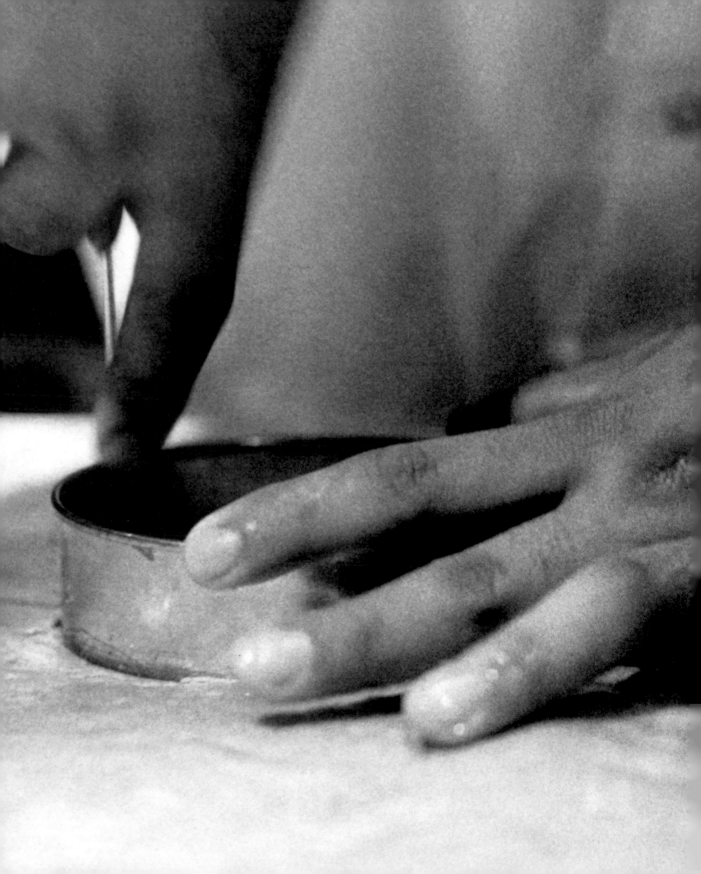

For the tomato-lime salsa:

3 cups finely chopped, seeded tomatoes
3 tablespoons lime juice
1 handful cilantro leaves, finely chopped
$1/2$ small jalapeño, seeded and finely chopped
$3/4$ teaspoon sea salt

In a medium bowl, combine the salsa ingredients and taste for seasoning.

For the assembly:

3 limes for garnish
1 cup Tart Sour Cream (page 303)

1 Lay the tortillas on a flat surface. Spread 1 heaping tablespoon of the spicy "beans" and tomato sauce mixture on each tortilla, leaving a very thin rim at the edges. Top with a heaping tablespoon of guacamole. Fold the sides up to form a taco shape. Repeat with the remaining tortillas.

2 Cut each lime in half lengthwise (if you cut just on either side of the core of each lime, the sections are much easier to squeeze). Place a lime slice on each plate. Lay three filled tortillas against the lime and each other on the plates.

3 Top each tortilla with a heaping tablespoon of tomato-lime salsa and a drizzle of "sour cream." As you eat them, squeeze a bit of the lime garnish on each one.

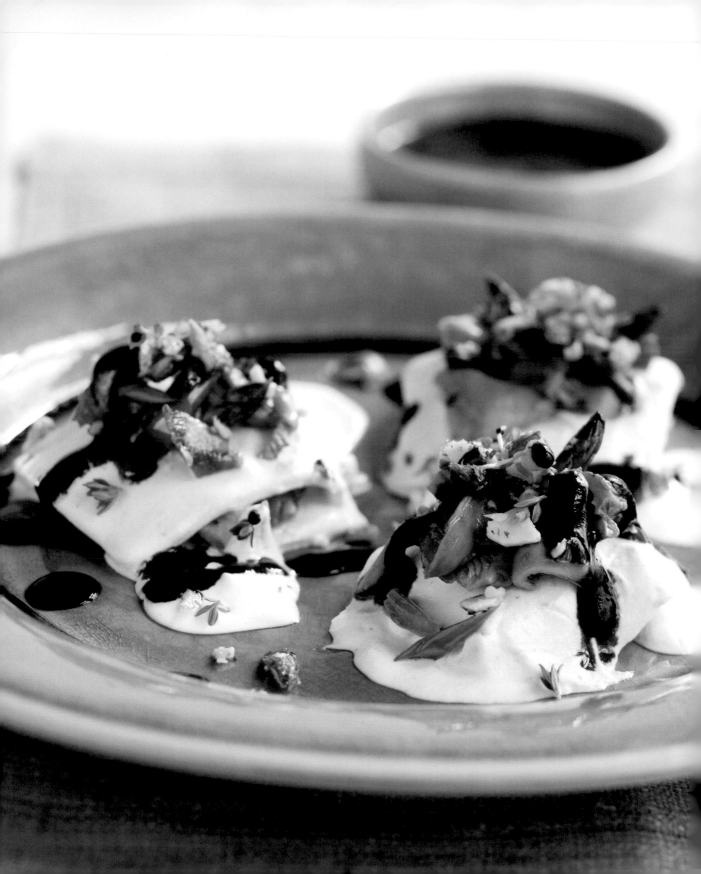

Asparagus and Porcini Ravioli

with lemon cream and balsamic-fig puree

SERVES 4

Cutting the coconuts in this recipe can be tricky. Some coconuts have very thick meat that is good for slicing, while the meat in others may be too thin and soft to use for this dish. (For how to properly cut coconuts, see page 64.) You may want to allow a few more coconuts for this reason. Save any of the too-soft meat to use in a shake or just eat it with a spoon! If you can't find fresh or dried figs, $1/2$ cup rehydrated raisins will work fine, or you can even just garnish the plate with a drizzle of plain, good quality balsamic vinegar.

Sarma and I were under pressure to come up with an interesting dish for our business partner, who was coming over for dinner. I was finishing up an intense yoga class when I began to envision this dish. To my surprise, it ended up exactly as I had imagined. It ultimately made it onto our restaurant menu, using wild asparagus and Meyer lemons when in season. —MK

For the asparagus and porcini filling:

1 small bunch thin asparagus
1/2 pound cleaned porcini mushrooms, or
    chanterelle, shiitake, or any
    combination of wild mushrooms*
3 tablespoons extra-virgin olive oil

3 tablespoons lemon juice
1 tablespoon fresh thyme
1 tablespoon minced fresh rosemary
Sea salt
Freshly ground black pepper

Cut the asparagus into 1/2-inch lengths, on a bias, discarding the woody ends. Cut the mushrooms into small pieces. In a medium bowl, toss the asparagus and mushrooms with the olive oil, lemon juice, thyme, and rosemary. Season with salt and pepper to taste. Spread out on a dehydrator sheet and dehydrate at 115°F for 2 to 3 hours, or until they are tender and taste like they've been sautéed.

Discard any unusable stems before measuring weight, so if you are using shiitakes, for example, you will probably need to purchase at least 3/4 pound.

For the lemon cream:

1 cup raw cashews, soaked for 2 hours
    or more
1 cup water
3 tablespoons lemon juice

1 tablespoon raw honey
1 tablespoon lemon zest
Sea salt

In a Vita-Mix or high-speed blender, puree the cashews, water, lemon juice, honey, and lemon zest until smooth. Add more water if needed for creamy sauce consistency. Season to taste with salt. Transfer the sauce to a bowl or covered container.

To make the balsamic-fig puree:

4 to 5 large fresh black mission figs, or
    rehydrated dried figs

1/2 cup high quality aged balsamic vinegar
Sea salt

In a Vita-Mix or high-speed blender, puree the figs and the balsamic vinegar until completely smooth. Season with salt and transfer to a squeeze bottle or covered container and set aside. Refrigerate if not using right away, for up to a few days.

For the assembly:

4 young coconuts (more or less depending on their yield)
1 small handful chopped raw almonds, preferably soaked and dehydrated
2 teaspoons almond oil or other cold-pressed oil
Coarse sea salt
Freshly ground black pepper
Baby chervil or other fine herbs for garnish (optional)

1 With a cleaver, chop the top off the young coconuts. Reserve or drink the coconut water. Using the back of a spoon, carefully remove the meat from the top and the inside of the coconut, trying to keep the meat in large pieces as much as possible when removing it (if the meat is too soft, use it for a shake, and try your luck with the next coconut!). Cut the meat into 2-inch squares and slice the squares lengthwise as thinly as possible with a very sharp filleting knife. You should have 24 squares. Save any coconut meat scraps for shakes. Set the coconut squares aside, or refrigerate if not using right away.

2 Dip the coconut ravioli squares in the lemon cream to coat well, and place three on each of 4 plates, at three points. Sauce the plates with the balsamic-fig puree so that some of the sauce will end up inside the raviolis. Top each coconut square with about a tablespoon of the mushroom and asparagus mixture and cover with another coconut square, also dipped in the sauce. Spoon a bit of the remaining lemon sauce over each ravioli. Top again with a bit of the mushroom and asparagus mixture.

3 In a small bowl, toss the chopped almonds with almond oil and season with coarse sea salt. Sprinkle each ravioli with the chopped almond mixture. Sprinkle with black pepper, and garnish with herbs, if desired.

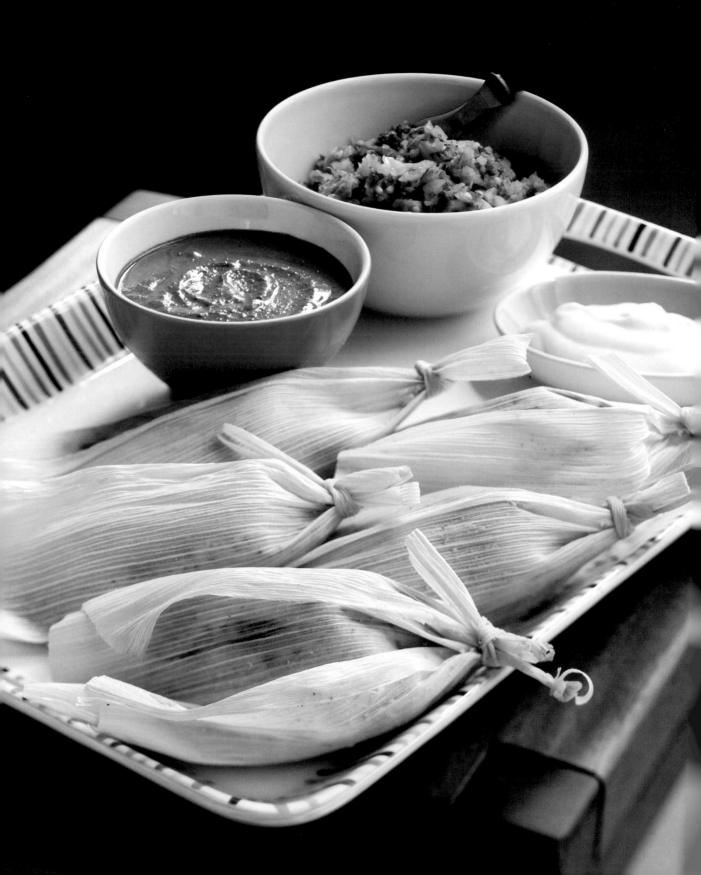

White Corn Tamales

with raw cacao mole, marinated portobellos, and green tomato salsa

SERVES 4 TO 6 (MAKES 12 TAMALES)

Traditionally, Mexican mole sauce is made like curry: ground chili peppers, spices, and flavorings are combined according to a cook's taste and intention. In this recipe, we use raw cacao beans, the unadulterated seeds of the cacao tree that are extremely rich in antioxidant flavenols, significantly more so than even red wine and green tea. We use both raw cacao and organic cocoa powder for a more balanced flavor. Green & Black's organic cocoa from the United Kingdom is the best brand to use but is not easy to find (see "Sources," page 358) Making the mole sauce can be hard on your blender, so it is best to use a Vita-Mix or one with a strong motor.

This is an impressive dish to serve guests—its presentation in the corn husk is rustic and fun. —MK

For the portobellos:

3 medium or 2 large portobello mushroom caps, sliced into sticks about 2 inches long and 1/4-inch thick

1/2 cup pumpkin seed oil
1 clove garlic, minced
1 tablespoon minced fresh oregano
1 teaspoon sea salt

In a medium bowl, toss the mushrooms with the pumpkin seed oil, garlic, oregano, and salt. Add a bit more oil if necessary to coat all the mushrooms. Transfer the mushrooms to a Teflex-lined dehydrator tray and dehydrate at 115°F for 12 to 24 hours (tossing them around from time to time) or until the mushrooms taste as if they have been sautéed.

For the mole sauce:

3 dried chili peppers (such as ancho,
      pasilla, or cascabel)
3 tablespoons raw cacao nibs
      (see Sources, page 358)
1/2 cup pumpkin seeds or sunflower seeds
1/4 cup sesame seeds

3/4 cup raisins
1/2 teaspoon cumin
1/4 cup raw almond butter
1 tablespoon cocoa powder
2 tablespoons walnut or other nut oil
Sea salt
Freshly ground black pepper

1 In a bowl, add the chilies, cacao nibs, pumpkin seeds, sesame seeds, raisins, and cumin and mix to combine. Add enough water to the bowl to cover and let stand at room temperature for 1 to 2 hours.

2 Transfer the mixture to a Vita-Mix or high-speed blender, add the almond butter and cocoa powder, and blend until completely smooth, adding as much filtered water as necessary to get it to a thick-sauce consistency. Add the walnut oil, and sea salt and black pepper to taste and blend to combine.

For the corn filling and tamales:

12 corn husks
6 cups fresh white corn kernels,
      cut from 4–5 ears
1 cup pine nuts

1 cup cashews
1/2 teaspoon cayenne
1 teaspoon sea salt
1 small handful cilantro, finely chopped

1 Soak the corn husks in warm water for 1 to 2 hours to make them pliable.

2 Place 5 cups of the corn in the food processor with the pine nuts, cashews, cayenne, and salt and process just until smooth, but do not overprocess. Fold in the remaining 1 cup corn and the cilantro and adjust seasoning if necessary. Transfer to a bowl and mix in the dehydrated mushrooms.

3 Dry the corn husks with a towel. Tear a thin strip off the side of each husk—this will be used as string to tie the tamale together. Lay the corn husks flat and place about ½ cup of the corn mixture onto the center of each. Fold the bottoms up over the filling and then fold the sides over. Using the husk strips, tie the tops of each tamale.

4 Place the tamales in the dehydrator at 115°F to warm them through, ideally for about 2 hours before serving.

For the salsa verde:

2 to 3 medium green tomatoes

2 to 3 medium tomatillos

Sea salt

2 jalapeño peppers, seeds to taste, chopped

1 very large handful cilantro

1 green onion, white and 1 inch green, chopped

2 tablespoons lime juice

Quarter and salt the tomatoes and tomatillos. Let sit for 1 hour and then drain the liquid and place them in the food processor. Add the jalapeño, cilantro, and green onion and pulse until chunky. Drain any additional excess liquid and discard, and season the mixture with lime juice and salt to taste.

For serving:

½ cup Tart Sour Cream (page 303)

Cocoa powder for dusting

Baby cilantro or regular cilantro for garnish

1 Spoon mole sauce onto each plate and spread to make a wide pool.

2 Using a sharp knife, carefully slice open the tamales and place 2 or 3 on top of the sauce on each plate. Gently pull the tamales open a bit and top each with a heaping tablespoon of salsa. Place a spoonful of sour cream on the mole sauce, dust the plate with cocoa powder, and garnish with cilantro.

Green Curry Coconut Noodles

with spring vegetables

We're not enthused about utilizing a prepackaged, premixed curry. Rather, we like to combine spices on our own—that way the curry is as individual as, well, the individual. We mix cumin and turmeric with smaller quantities of spices such as cardamom, cinnamon, ginger, and mustard seed. But if you prefer, you can use a high-quality mix and/or add more quantities of any spice to taste.

I like the textures in this dish—crunchy vegetables with smooth and slippery noodles. The umeboshi and miso make the vegetables a bit sweet while the sauce is nice and spicy.   —MK

For the spring vegetables:

3 tablespoons umeboshi plum paste (see Sources, page 362)
$^1/_4$ cup extra-virgin olive oil
$^1/_4$ cup white miso
3 tablespoons brown rice vinegar
2 tablespoons chopped ginger
2 teaspoons sesame oil
2 green onions, white and 1 inch green, one coarsely chopped, the other thinly sliced on a bias
1 cup thinly sliced yellow squash, cut into $^1/_8$-inch-thick half-moons)
1 cup thinly sliced zucchini (cut into $^1/_8$-inch-thick half-moons)
1 cup chanterelles, cut in pieces
1 small carrot, cut into thin matchsticks
1 cup sliced snap peas, cut on bias into diamond shapes
1 small stalk celery, cut in half lengthwise and then cut on bias into thin slices

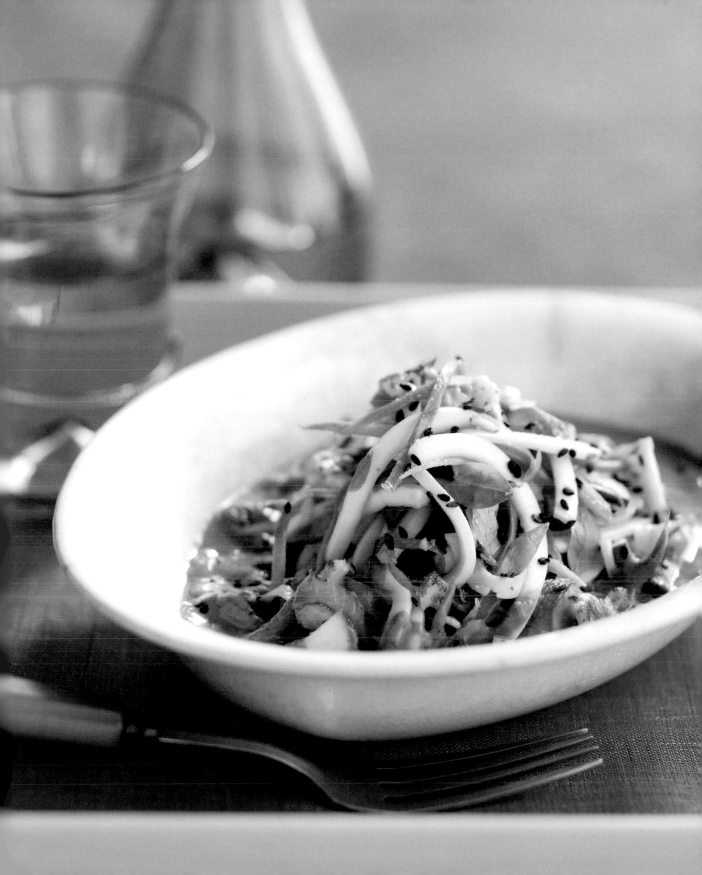

In a blender, puree the plum paste, olive oil, miso, brown rice vinegar, ginger, sesame oil, and the coarsely chopped green onion until smooth. Add the thinly sliced green onion to all of the remaining ingredients in a medium bowl. Add the plum paste sauce to the vegetables and toss to coat. Set aside to marinate at room temperature for 1 to 4 hours, or place in the refrigerator if keeping longer, up to 1 day.

For the green curry:

$^1/_4$ cup grated lemongrass

1 cup coconut meat

$^1/_4$ cup raw cashew nuts, soaked
for 1 hour or more

2 tablespoons lime juice

3 tablespoons chopped jalapeño,
seeds to taste

3 green onions, white and 1 inch green

2 tablespoons chopped ginger

$^1/_4$ cup loosely packed basil

About 2 teaspoons curry powder

1 teaspoon sea salt

$^1/_4$ cup coconut water

Lemongrass can be chopped and then blended in if using a Vita-Mix. Place all of the green curry ingredients, except the coconut water, in a blender and puree. Add the coconut water a bit at a time until a thick-sauce consistency is achieved.

For serving:

$^1/_2$ cup chopped raw almonds, preferably
soaked and dehydrated

1 teaspoon sesame oil

$^1/_2$ teaspoon sea salt

2 cups coconut noodles, from about 4
coconuts (see page 64 on making
coconut noodles)

1 large handful cilantro, coarsely chopped

1 small handful mint, coarsely chopped or torn

1 small handful basil, coarsely chopped or torn

2 tablespoons black sesame seeds

1 In a small bowl, toss the almonds with the sesame oil and salt.

2 Add the coconut noodles to the spring vegetables, add the herbs, and toss to combine. Divide the vegetables and noodles among serving plates. Spoon the curry around the noodles. Sprinkle with the chopped almonds and black sesame seeds.

Raw Cacao

Chocolate-loving raw foodist? No, it's not an oxymoron. Chocolate, or cacao, does not have to be dried, roasted, processed, and mixed with dried milk solids to be tasty. Essentially, raw cacao beans are bittersweet chocolate, tasting like unsweetened baking chocolate, and they are to the brain what blueberries are to the body—a superfood. Containing more than 300 chemicals, many of them resembling our natural brain lipids, raw cacao has so many healing and feel-good properties that even mass-market candy companies are beginning to add it to their commercial, cooked products. Happy pills, indeed! For the raw food community, sweetening ground raw cacao with a little agave nectar is the base for many shakes, smoothies, and soul-satisfying desserts (see Sources, page 358).

Umeboshi Plums

Umeboshi are Japanese pickled plums (*ume*), also known as salt plums. The fruit is picked green, then cured in brine and red shiso leaves, which tinge the plums (just as red grape skins give their color to wine), anywhere from pink to ruby. The taste is both unique and complex, with sweet, sour, tart, and salty elements, and the texture is baby-soft. Umoboshi can be pureed into a paste, concentrated into a syrup, or eaten out-of-hand—try one with a cocktail instead of a chemically treated olive or pickled onion! The paste is a terrific seasoning agent, and because *ume* have the highest levels of citric acid of any fruit, which help break down lactic acid and cleanse the body, they're also extremely good for fighting fatigue and slowing down the dreaded aging process. Be wary of the nonraw concentrate, though, as it's made by boiling down the plums. You can find umeboshi plums and umeboshi plum vinegar in most health food and ethnic stores (see Sources, page 362).

Cauliflower Samosas

with banana tamarind sauce, mango chutney, and mint

SERVES 4 (ABOUT 20 SAMOSAS)

Samosas—deep-fried vegetarian turnovers—are a classic Indian street food. Our version is a bit more delicate than the fried variety, but incredibly savory. You can make them a few hours ahead and keep them warming on trays in the dehydrator; this also keeps them dry, so they won't stick together, as they would if you piled them up and set them aside. They are a perfect hors d'oeuvre, or you could serve just a few of them per plate as a starter.

This recipe calls for Chunky Chat masala, a very cool ingredient that you can find at most Indian stores. It's very tasty and we also just like saying "Chunky Chat." If you can't find it, simply substitute more garam masala and call it a day. One of our ever-resourceful chefs, Glory, who worked previously at the very highly regarded New York City Indian restaurant, Tabla, found out what exactly is in it. *Chat* means 'to lick' and 'masala' means 'blend of ground spices.' Chunky Chat masala generally contains green mango powder, smoky black salt, cumin, and asafoetida, as well as other spices. While we're at it, garam masala (garam means 'warming') contains coriander seed, cumin, cardamom, black pepper, cloves, cinnamon, and nutmeg. Now, I suspect that some of those spices may have been toasted, and therefore are not 100 percent raw, but I wouldn't be too concerned about a tiny amount of spice here and there. Life, even on a raw diet, is still too short for that. —SM

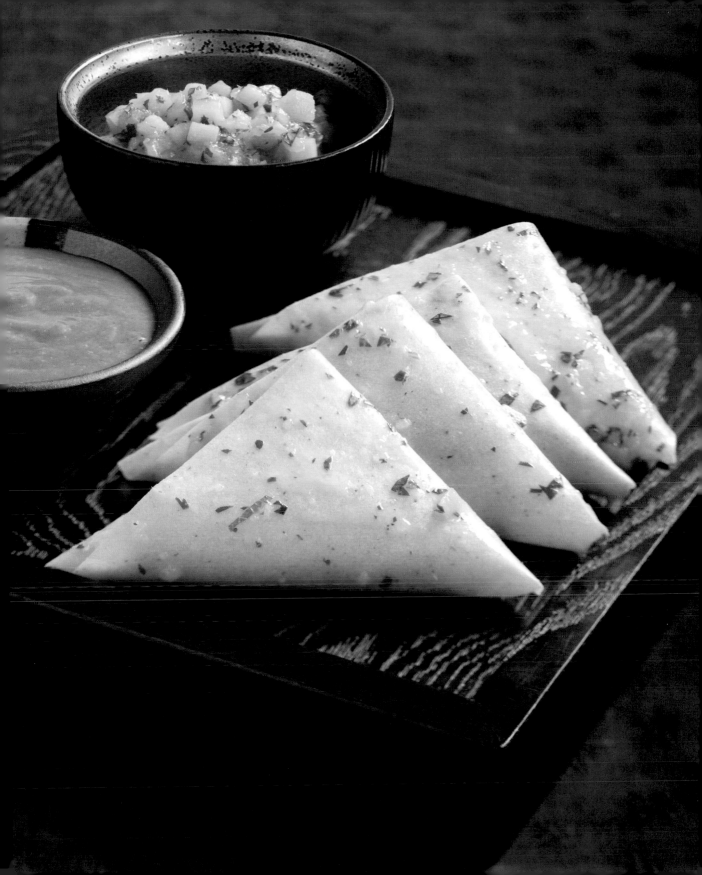

For the samosa wraps:

2 cups young coconut meat
1½ cups coconut water (or more)
½ teaspoon cayenne
½ teaspoon sea salt

1 In a Vita-Mix or high-speed blender, puree the coconut with the coconut water, cayenne, and salt until completely smooth. Using an offset spatula, spread the coconut *very* thin on Teflex-lined dehydrator trays and dehydrate at 115°F for 2 to 4 hours, or until the surface is dry. Carefully flip over and peel away the Teflex sheets. Dehydrate further on the screen only, just to dry the underside, 15 to 30 minutes longer. The wraps should be very thin, almost transparent, and very pliable.

2 Carefully slide the wraps onto a flat cutting surface and cut into large rectangles, about 3 by 7 inches, and set aside.

For the filling:

1 large head cauliflower, florets only
½ cup raw macadamia nuts
1 cup filtered water
1 tablespoon garam masala
2 teaspoons Chunky Chat masala (or substitute garam masala)
1 tablespoon chopped fresh ginger
Sea salt
Freshly ground black pepper
1 cup fresh peas or thawed frozen peas
1 handful julienned cilantro

1 Place the cauliflower florets in a food processor and pulse a few times to chop into small pieces. It's okay if they are not entirely uniform in size—they add texture.

2 In a Vita-Mix or high-speed blender, add the nuts, water, garam masala, Chunky Chat, and ginger and puree at high speed for 2 minutes until completely smooth. It should be the consistency of heavy cream. Season with salt and pepper to taste.

3 Add the cauliflower, peas, and macadamia cream to a shallow glass bowl or pan and stir to combine. Place the bowl in the dehydrator and dehydrate at 115°F for about 2 hours, stirring occasionally, until the cauliflower becomes somewhat tender and the cream thickens a bit.

4 Toss the cilantro in with the cauliflower mixture just before filling the wraps.

For the banana tamarind sauce:

1 cup Tamarind Sauce (page 145)
1 small banana
1 teaspoon ground cumin
1 teaspoon minced ginger
1 small red chili pepper, seeded
Pinch of sea salt

Puree the sauce ingredients in a blender until completely smooth. Transfer to a separate container and set aside.

For serving:

1 cup Mango Chutney (page 301)
1 small handful mint leaves, finely julienned

1 Place a heaping tablespoon of cauliflower filling at one end of a coconut wrapper. Fold one corner over diagonally to meet the other side, to form a triangle. Fold the samosa over and continue folding like a flag. Wet the end of the wrapper slightly to seal.

2 Serve the samosa with the mango chutney and the banana tamarind sauce and sprinkle with fresh mint.

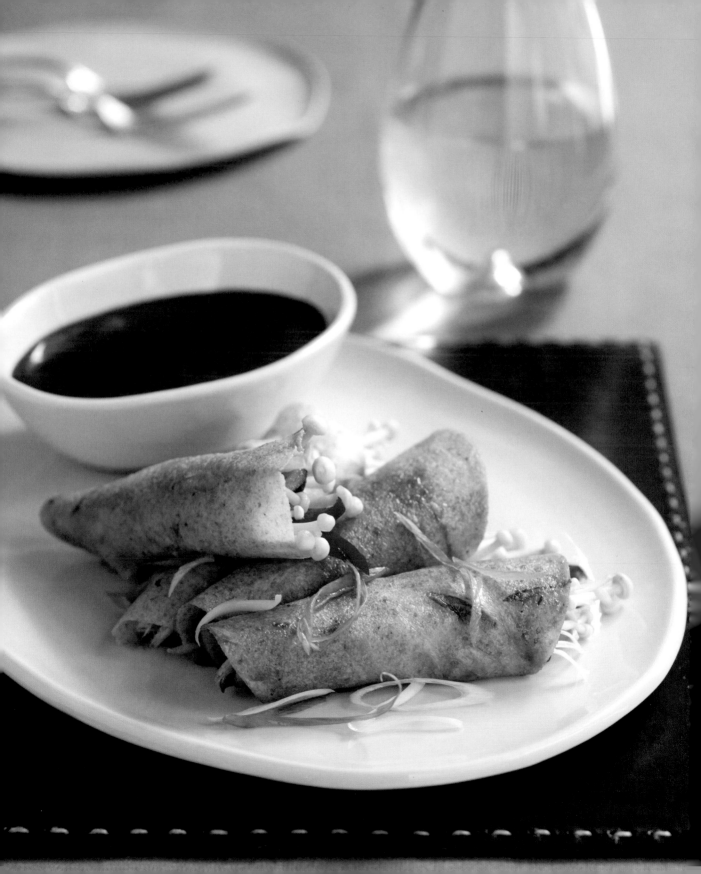

Japanese Eggplant-Filled Scallion Pancake

with black bean sauce and plum hoisin

SERVES 4

Red flesh plums will make a beautiful, dark pink sauce, but any kind will do. Fermented black soybeans can be found in any Asian market or in the Asian section of some health food stores or supermarkets.

> "This recipe was the creation of one of our sous-chefs, Louisa, and it was Donna Karan's favorite dish when she first came to the restaurant. Because it's one of the few more complex dishes that contain absolutely no nuts, it's good for people who have the much-dreaded nut allergy." —MK

For the pancakes:

4 cups coconut meat

$1^1/_3$ cups diced yellow squash

1 cup filtered water

1 cup flaxseeds, finely ground
(about $1^1/_3$ cup ground)

$^1/_2$ cup thinly sliced scallion,
white and 1 inch green

2 to 3 teaspoons salt

2 Thai chilies, minced

$^1/_4$ cup sesame oil

1 In a Vita-Mix or high-speed blender, blend the coconut meat with the yellow squash, adding water $^1/_4$ cup at a time as needed to make it smooth. You may need to use the tamper (the large, black, baton-like thing that comes with your Vita-Mix) to push the squash and coconut into the blades. The resulting mixture should be thick, like a custard.

2 Transfer the coconut mixture to a large bowl and add the flaxseeds, scallions, and salt. Mix it very thoroughly with a spatula or large spoon.

3 Divide the batter between three 14-inch Teflex-lined dehydrator trays. Using an offset spatula, spread to about $^1/_6$-inch thickness and sprinkle with the minced Thai chiles. Dehydrate at 115°F for 6 to 8 hours or overnight. Flip them over and peel away the Teflex. Continue dehydrating on the screens only for another hour or two, until the underside is just dry and the pancake is still pliable.

4 Slide the pancake sheet onto a cutting surface and brush with sesame oil. Using a circle cutter (or you can trace around a small plate with a sharp knife), cut circles about 4 inches in diameter. You should get 6 round pancakes per tray, for a total of 18 pancakes.

For the filling:

3 cups Japanese eggplant, cut in half and
    then on a bias into half-moons
2 teaspoons fine sea salt
$^1/_3$ cup fermented black beans
$^1/_4$ cup plus 3 tablespoons sesame oil
$^1/_4$ cup plus 3 tablespoons nama shoyu

$^1/_4$ cup plus 3 tablespoons maple syrup
$^1/_4$ cup plus 3 tablespoons ginger juice
3 cups thinly sliced red, purple, or yellow
    bell peppers, cut into 1-inch lengths
2 cups trimmed and sliced yellow wax beans,
    cut into $^1/_2$-half-inch lengths on a bias

1 In a medium bowl, toss the eggplant with the salt, let sit for 30 minutes until juices are released. Rinse the eggplant and squeeze out the excess liquid. Place the eggplant in a medium bowl with the black beans and 3 tablespoons each of sesame oil, nama shoyu, maple syrup, and ginger juice and toss to combine. Transfer to a shallow bowl or container and place in dehydrator for about 6 hours at 115°F, stirring occasionally, until tender.

2 In a medium bowl, toss the peppers and the wax beans with the remaining $^1/_4$ cup each of sesame oil, nama shoyu, maple syrup, and ginger juice. Dehydrate at 115°F for about 2 hours, or until tender.

For the plum hoisin sauce:

2 cups sliced fresh plums
$\frac{1}{2}$ cup sesame oil
$\frac{1}{2}$ cup mirin
$\frac{1}{4}$ cup nama shoyu
$\frac{1}{2}$ cup maple syrup
$\frac{1}{2}$ cup ginger juice
Sea salt

1 Dehydrate the sliced plums on a dehydrator screen at 115°F for 8 to 10 hours, or overnight.

2 In a Vita-Mix or high-speed blender, blend the dehydrated plums, sesame oil, mirin, nama shoyu, maple syrup, and ginger juice until smooth. Pass through a fine-mesh strainer, and season with additional salt, if necessary. Place in a squeeze bottle or other covered container.

For serving:

1 bunch enoki mushrooms, solid end sliced off but stems left long
2 green onions, thinly sliced on a bias, or minced chives or whole micro-herbs, for garnish

1 In a medium bowl, combine the eggplant, peppers, and wax beans and keep warm in the dehydrator before serving. To serve, lay the pancakes flat and place about 2 heaping tablespoons of the vegetable mixture in the center of each. Lay a few of the enoki mushrooms on top of each and carefully roll up.

2 Sauce each of the plates with hoisin. Divide the rolled pancakes among the plates and garnish with the green onions.

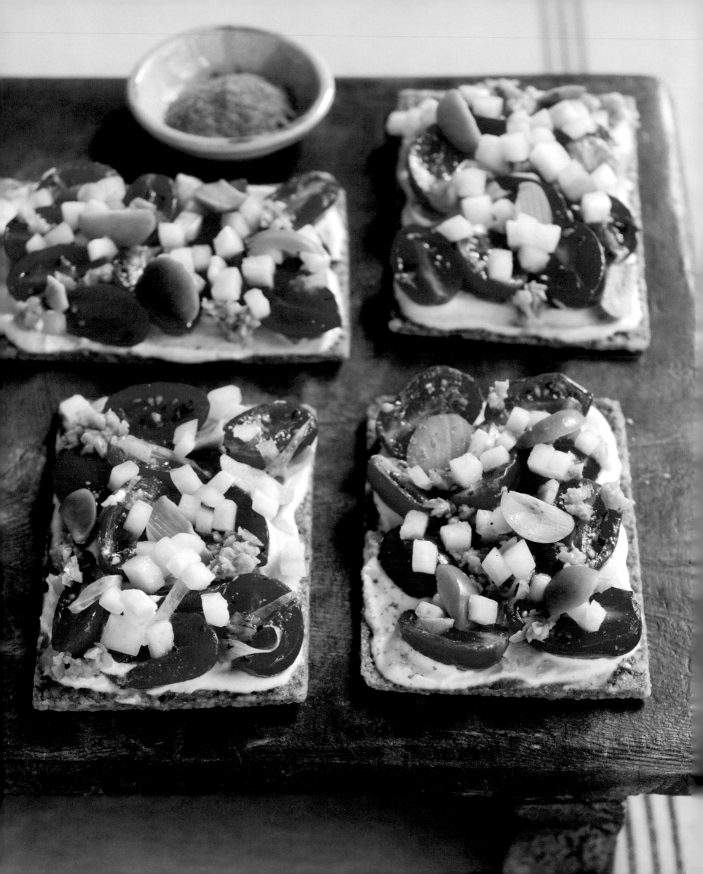

Flatbread Pizza

with hummus, green olives, cherry tomatoes, and za'atar

SERVES 4 TO 6

Za'atar is a ubiquitous Middle-Eastern spice blend used to season everything from olives to meatballs. It is comprised of lemony sumac, nutty sesame seeds, and the wild Syrian hyssop plant, an herb similar in aroma and essence to thyme or oregano. Each country has its own version, therefore you can find reasonable, prepacked approximations of it in markets ranging from Israeli to Lebanese. You can also make your own to spec, as with curry—check the Web for a variety of recipes.

> " The key to making this dish successfully is keeping the crust thin and crispy, so as not to overwhelm the delicate flavors of the fresh ingredients. This pizza was influenced generally by our love for the Mediterranean and specifically by a flatbread pizza with za'atar that we tried at a friend's restaurant. Its fresh, lemony flavor is a great counterpart to the sweet tomatoes, crunchy fennel, and salty olives. " —MK

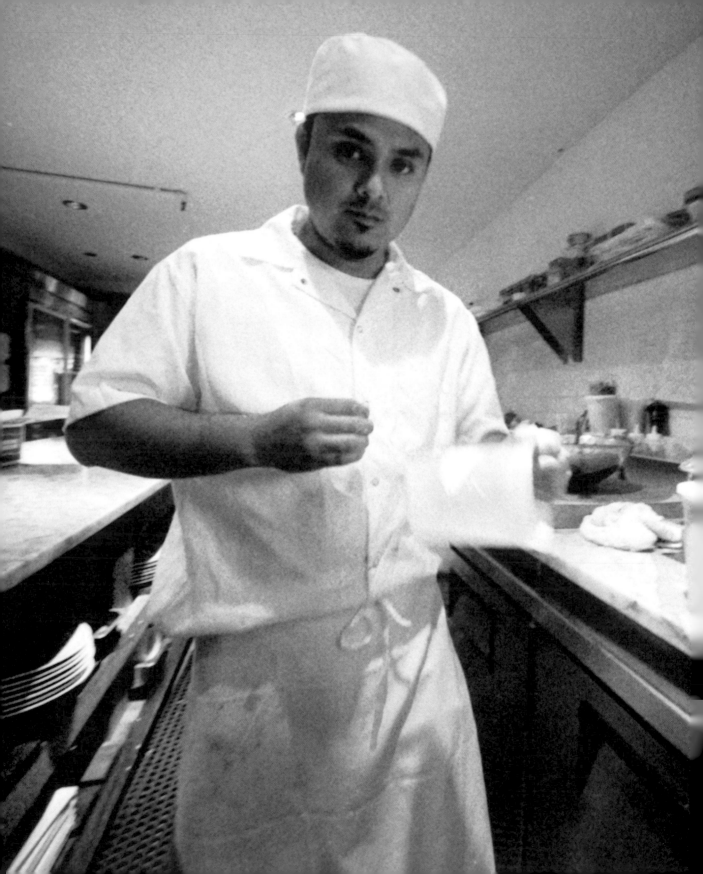

For the crusts:

5 cups walnuts, soaked 1 hour or more
5 cups cubed yellow squash or zucchini
³/₄ cup golden flaxseed, finely ground (1 cup ground)
¹/₂ cup hemp seeds
¹/₄ to ¹/₂ cup filtered water
1 tablespoon sea salt

1 Pulse the walnuts in a food processor to chop into tiny pieces (like couscous), but not completely smooth. Transfer the nuts to a large bowl. Add the squash to the same food processor bowl and grind into tiny pieces, but again not completely smooth. Transfer the squash to the bowl with the walnuts. Add the flaxseed, hemp seeds, salt, and about ¹/₄ cup of water, stirring to combine. Add more water until a sticky dough forms—like wet muffin batter. You may need more or less water.

2 Divide the batter between four 14-inch Teflex-lined dehydrator trays. Using an offset spatula, spread the dough to the edges of the trays. The dough can be a bit gummy and sticky, so it helps to dip the spatula in water as you spread the dough (the excess water will all evaporate in the dehydrator).

3 Dehydrate the flatbread at 115°F for 6 to 8 hours, or overnight. When the tops are dry, flip them over and peel away the Teflex liners. Dehydrate on screens for another 2 to 4 hours.

4 Once both sides are dry, slide the flatbread onto a large cutting board. With a large chef's knife, cut into 3 by 5-inch rectangles (or whatever size and shape you want). Place them back on the dehydrator trays and dehydrate another hour or more, as necessary for firm crusts.

For the hummus:

4 cups cashews, soaked for 2 hours or more
$^1/_2$ cup lemon juice
2 small cloves garlic
$^1/_4$ cup sesame tahini
1 teaspoon sea salt
1 cup filtered water

In a food processor, add the nuts, lemon juice, garlic, tahini, and salt and process, adding water $^1/_4$ cup at a time until you get the smooth, fluffy consistency of hummus. You may need to add more water, or you may want to add olive oil for a richer hummus—just make sure it has enough stiffness so it will hold the toppings on the pizza without running off the sides of the crust.

For serving:

1 pint cherry, teardrop, or grape tomatoes, halved
$^1/_4$ of a large bulb of fennel, or $^1/_2$ of a small bulb, shaved very thin on a mandoline
$^1/_2$ English cucumber, peeled, seeded, and finely diced
$^1/_2$ cup Green Olive Tapenade (page 302)
$^1/_2$ cup green olives, pitted and halved
2 tablespoons za'atar seasoning
Fennel fronds for garnish

Spread each crust with hummus and top with tomatoes, fennel, cucumber, olive tapenade, and olives. Sprinkle with the za'atar and top with fennel fronds.

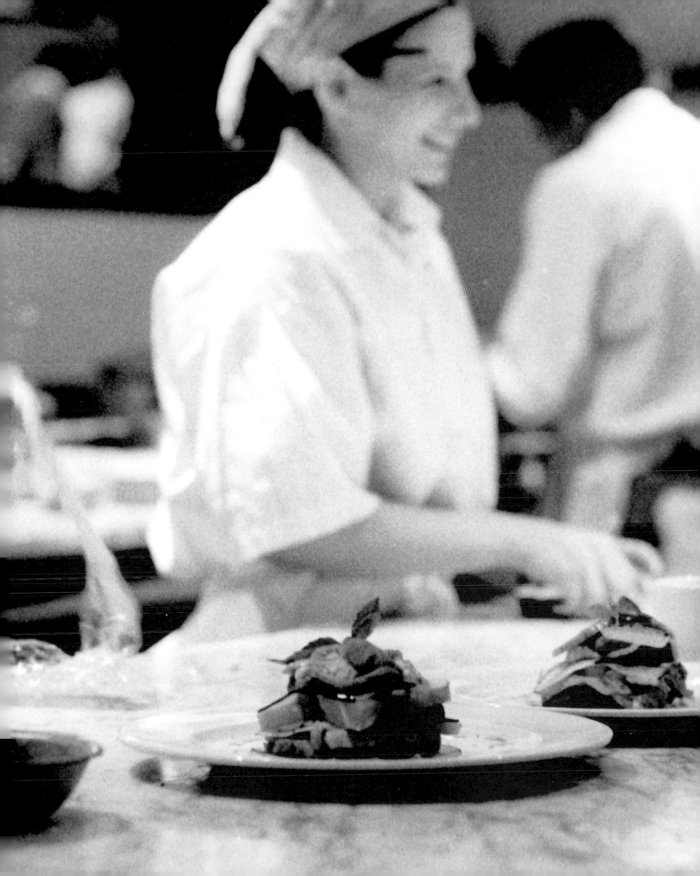

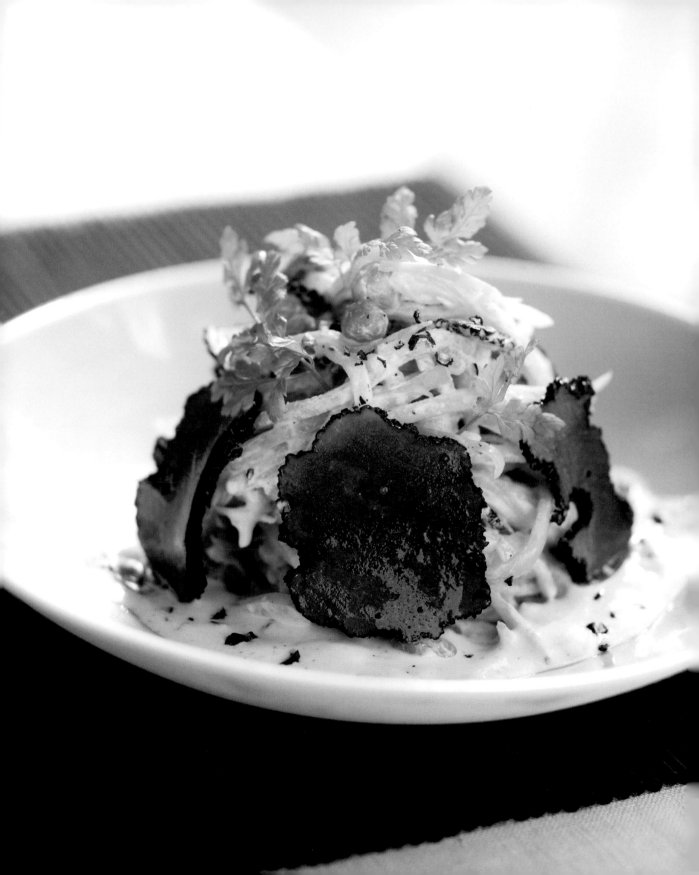

Golden Squash Pasta

with black summer truffles, creamy truffle sauce, and sweet peas

SERVES 4

We've nothing against the white variety of truffles (except maybe the price!). Black summer truffles, which are harvested earlier in the year than the white Piemontese sort, are less expensive and have a more modest pungency. They can be purchased online or at high-end specialty stores. If they're out of season, use a bit more of the truffle paste, which comes in a jar and might be pasteurized; though technically not raw, at less than a teaspoon per serving we think it can squeeze by the raw food police. Try a bit of truffle oil if you can't locate the paste.

For the sauce:

1 cup chopped celery root

1/2 medium sweet-tart apple, such as Fuji

1 cup raw cashews,
    soaked 4 hours or more

3 tablespoons lemon juice

1 tablespoon nutritional yeast

About 1 tablespoon truffle paste
    (see Sources, page 366)

Sea salt

Freshly ground black pepper

In a juicer, juice the celery root and the apple and add both to a Vita-Mix or high-speed blender with the cashews, lemon juice, and yeast. Blend until completely smooth, adding water if necessary to thin it to a creamy sauce consistency. Add the truffle paste, salt, and pepper, to taste.

For serving:

2 to 3 medium goldbar squash,
   julienned on a mandoline
Sea salt
1 small black summer truffle,
   shaved thin on a mandoline (see
   Sources, page 366)

½ pint freshly shelled peas
½ bunch chives, cut in small batons
Freshly ground black pepper
2 teaspoons hazelnut or truffle oil
1 squeeze lemon juice
Chervil blossoms, or fresh chervil leaves

1 Place the squash in a colander, toss with about ½ teaspoon sea salt, and let sit for at least 30 minutes to allow a bit of the liquid to drain out.

2 Place the squash in a medium bowl. Finely julienne about half of the truffle slices and add to the squash along with the peas and chives. Add a ladleful or two of sauce—enough to lightly coat the squash—season with pepper and toss.

3 Divide the squash pasta among 4 shallow serving bowls and spoon the remaining sauce around it. In a small bowl, toss the remaining truffle slices with the oil, lemon juice, and a pinch of sea salt. Arrange the slices around the pasta. Garnish with the chervil.

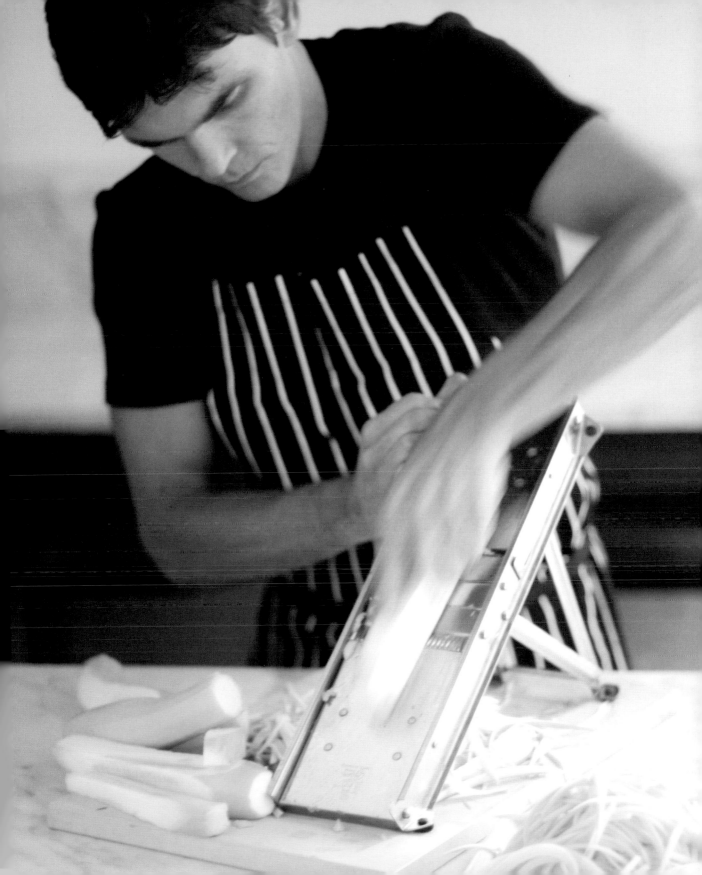

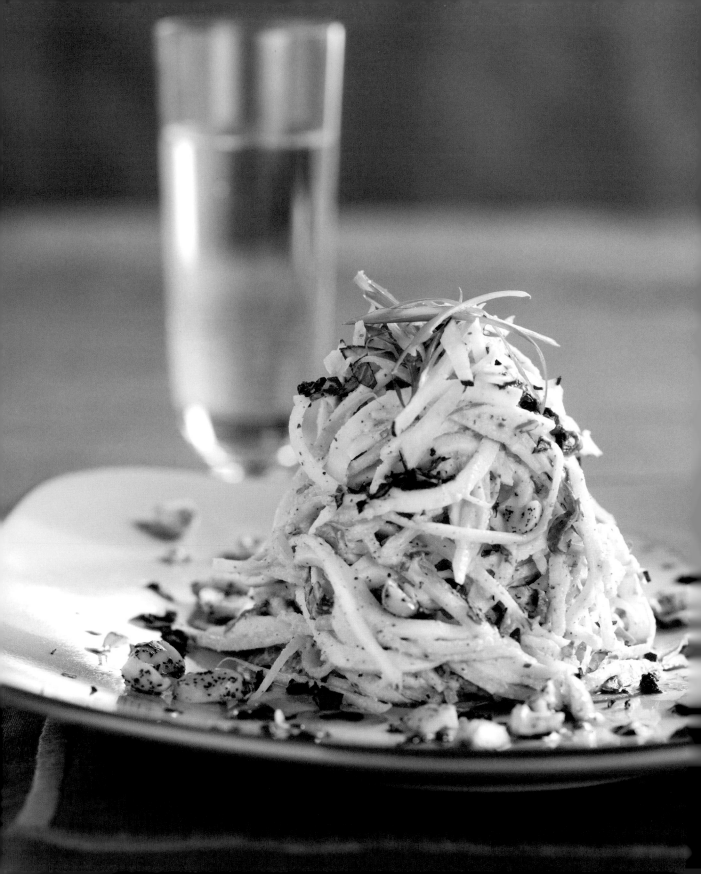

Spicy Peanut Coconut Noodles

with ginger and lime

SERVES 4

Peanuts are technically a legume, although you wouldn't necessarily think so considering someone misleadingly named them "pea*nuts*." Make sure you get really fresh, organically grown peanuts. Some debate persists about peanuts having toxicity, but it seems this may be from peanuts that are too old; at any rate, most toxins and other undesirables are washed away in the soaking process. However, if you don't feel comfortable eating peanuts, try this with cashews.

> One of our chefs, Amanda, helped us turn this idea into a really great, flavorful dish. The flesh of young Thai coconuts makes perfect noodles—although they are soft, they do not stick together and are as easy or easier to eat than regular starchy noodles. —MK

For the spiced peanuts:

1¹/₄ cups raw peanuts, coarsely chopped and soaked 4 hours or more
¹/₄ cup raw honey
2 teaspoons ground chili pepper
¹/₂ teaspoon sea salt

Drain and dry the peanuts and toss them in a medium bowl with the honey, chili pepper, and salt until well coated. Spread them in one layer on a Teflex-lined dehydrator tray and dehydrate at 115°F for 1 to 2 days, until crunchy.

For the peanut sauce:

¹/₃ cup coconut meat

1 cup coconut water

2 cups peanuts, soaked 4 hours or more

¹/₄ cup nama shoyu

1 cup chopped ginger

¹/₂ cup galangal

³/₄ cup raw almond butter

2 small red chili peppers, seeds optional

¹/₂ to 1 cup filtered water

3 tablespoons maple syrup

¹/₂ cup lime juice

In a Vita-Mix or high-speed blender, blend all the sauce ingredients except the lime juice until smooth. If using right away, add the lime juice and blend further to combine. If not, store the sauce in a covered container in the refrigerator for up to 2 days. Before serving, bring to room temperature and thoroughly stir or blend in the lime juice to thin it out again.

For serving:

2 cups coconut noodles, from about
4 coconuts (page 64)

1 cup julienned jicama

1 cup julienned green papaya
(or green mango)

1 cup julienned bok choy

1 cup julienned French radishes

2 green onions, white and 1 inch green,
thinly sliced on a bias

1 large handful cilantro

1 small handful Thai basil

1 tablespoon finely minced red chili pepper

Coarse sea salt

2 tablespoons sesame oil

2 tablespoons nama shoyu

2 limes, cut in half

In a large bowl, add the coconut noodles, jicama, green papaya, and the peanut sauce and toss to coat well. Add the bok choy, radishes, green onions, cilantro, half of the basil, half of the red chile, a sprinkle of salt, and gently toss. Divide among 4 serving plates and sprinkle with the spiced peanuts and the remaining basil and chili. Drizzle the sesame oil and nama shoyu on the plate around the noodles and garnish with the lime halves (which should be squeezed over the noodles just before eating).

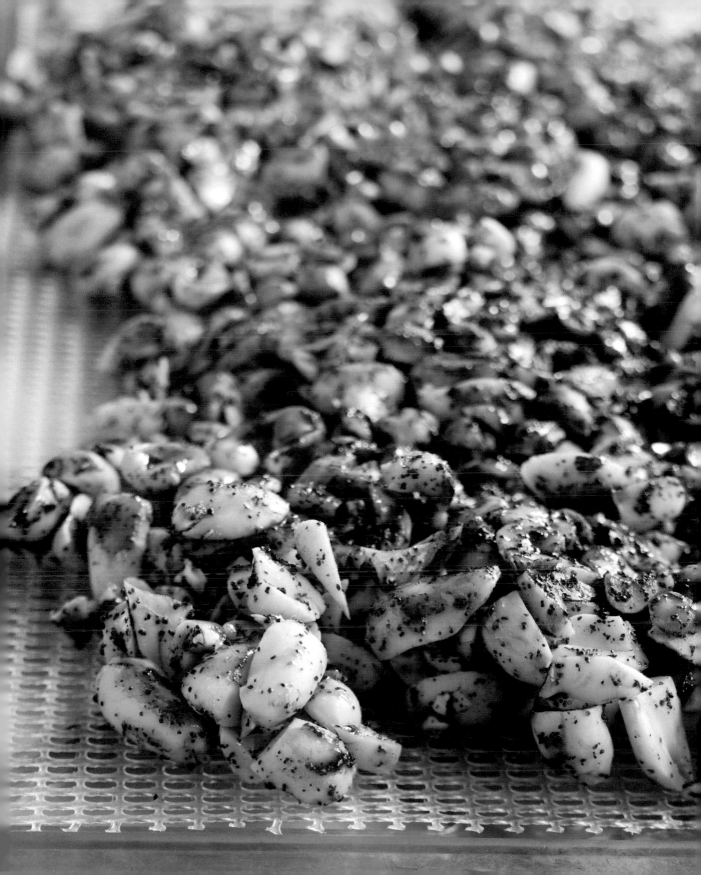

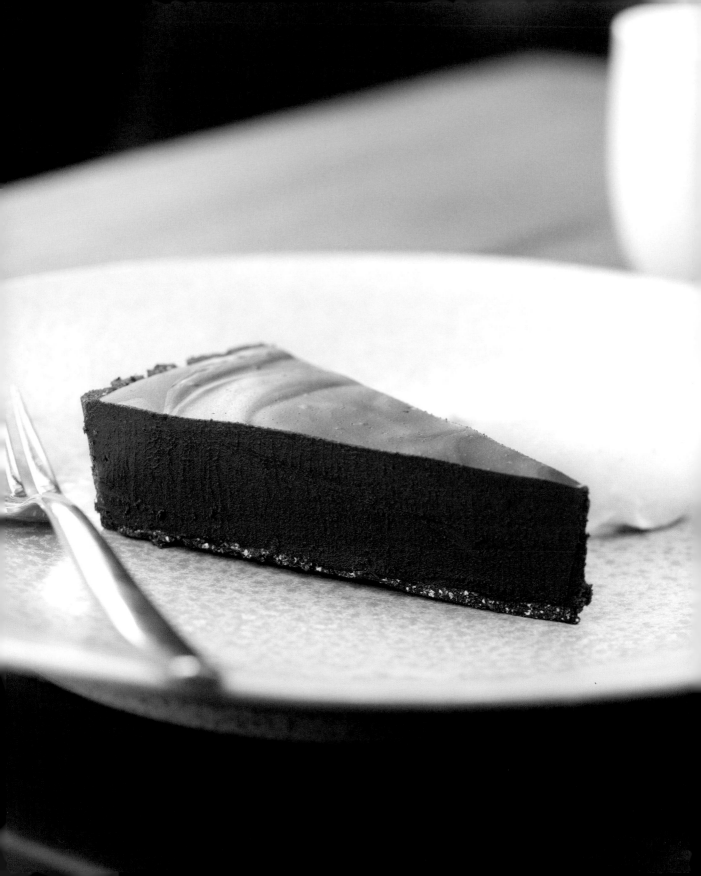

DESSERTS AND SWEETS

Desserts should make people happy. We have always loved lingering over something sweet at the end of a meal, though quite often sweets and desserts have been associated with guilt—something sinful only to be indulged in occasionally. We are now fortunate to have discovered that we can eat ice cream, cookies, tarts, and all of our other favorite treats—without gaining weight, facing sugar highs and lows, dealing with bad skin, headaches, mood swings, or any of the other side effects that come from eating refined sugar, white flour, eggs, and butter. Sharing a pint of ice cream from the restaurant at night is something we do all the time, and we feel happy about it!

We base most of our desserts on seasonal fruits and herbs. Although our popular chocolate tart is on our restaurant's menu year-round, we change nearly all the others throughout the year. We live and work within blocks of New York City's Union Square Greenmarket, which offers us an abundant choice of fruits in season, ranging from wild strawberries, white nectarines and peaches, apricots, gooseberries, sugar-plums, and blueberries in the summer to apples, pears, and concord grapes in the fall. We have made sauces, sorbets, tarts, and ice cream using all of these and more, and are constantly experimenting with new ways to "uncook" sweets.

We try to offer desserts that are satiating, not stupefying. After eating a meal at our restaurant, guests shouldn't feel full to the point of being tired or uncomfortable. The good news is, because all the ingredients are raw, you won't feel that way. Being able to eat a full meal, topping it off with a substantial dessert, and then getting up from the table and feeling like you want to go dancing all night are both the physiology and the psychology behind the raw food lifestyle.

At the restaurant, we pass all the custards through a fine-mesh strainer after blending to ensure that they are completely free of lumps or bumps. At home, where we only have ourselves to impress, we never bother with this step, so we have left it out of the recipes here. But if you're a perfectionist, strain away!

When working with coconut butter in desserts, it's important that the other ingredients are at room temperature. If they are too cold, the coconut butter might solidify into tiny solids that become difficult to incorporate.

Dessert Basics

Date paste: For desserts, we tend to use date paste rather than whole dates, which can be different sizes, as we can obtain more accurate measurements that way. The paste is also a convenient sweetener to have on hand, and can be used in smoothies or spread like jam. To make date paste: Soak pitted dates in water for 1 to 2 hours. Drain and reserve the water. Process the dates in a food processor, adding the soak water 1 tablespoon at a time as needed, until you have the consistency of a thick jam or butter. Transfer to a covered container and keep refrigerated. This should keep easily for a week, or much longer if frozen.

Almond flour: To make almond flour, soak almonds in water for at least 6 hours to overnight. Drain and rinse well and dehydrate for 12 hours. Pulse the almonds in a food processor for a fine consistency, but be careful not to overprocess (you don't want almond butter). Strain the almonds through a strainer to separate out the coarser pieces, leaving behind a fine almond flour. Some recipes call for the more coarse almond flour. You can keep both for future use, in covered containers, in the refrigerator for up to a week, or store longer in the freezer. You can also make the fine almond flour by dehydrating the pulp left behind when you make almond milk, however, in our experience it seems to go rancid rather quickly, so we don't recommend it.

Vanilla beans: Where we call for the seeds of fresh vanilla beans, split them in half lengthwise with the tip of a sharp paring knife, and scrape the seeds out with the edge of the knife. Generally one discards the pod, although a Vita-Mix can pulverize them quite well, and so we often save the pods to throw into shakes where they would get blended thoroughly. Vanilla beans, particularly the organic variety, are quite expensive. If you prefer not to buy them or can't find them, you can generally substitute about 2 teaspoons of vanilla extract per half vanilla bean in any recipe.

Maple syrup powder: Mostly used to make instant reconstituted syrup, maple syrup powder is a good sweetener in its own right. It can be difficult to find (see Sources, page 360) and remember, maple syrup products are not truly raw. If you use it just make sure it's pure and organic. For substitution guidelines for maple, see page 36.

Dark Chocolate Ganache Tart

with vanilla cream

Ganache, in traditional pastry terminology, refers to a mixture of cream and melted chocolate, sometimes tempered with butter. Using coconut butter instead, this version goes from artery clogging to heart healthy (see page 68 for benefits of coconut butter). You can substitute raw carob powder for the cocoa to make a carob tart, which is also good. However, we don't recommend substituting agave for the maple syrup in this dessert—it won't come out quite right. So if you are a more vigilant sort of raw foodist, you might want to leave this one out of your repertoire, but you'll be missing out!

Keep the tart chilled until serving—if you let it sit out at room temperature too long it will soften and start to melt, especially in warmer weather.

> This rich tart, a creation of Debbie Lee, our opening pastry chef, tastes almost sinful. It is one of the more popular desserts on our menu—I like the components as much as the whole. Try crumbling the crust mixture into some coconut or vanilla raw ice cream. —MK

For the tart crust:

³/₄ cup cocoa powder

³/₄ cup fine almond flour (page 230)

¹/₂ cup maple syrup powder (see Sources, page 360)

¹/₄ cup coconut butter

Pinch of sea salt

In a standing mixer with a paddle attachment, mix all the crust ingredients until thoroughly combined into a dough. You can do this by hand as well, with a wooden spoon in a large bowl. Press the dough evenly into a 9-inch tart pan with a removable bottom. Cover with plastic wrap and place in the refrigerator to chill 1 hour or more.

For the ganache filling:

2¼ cups cocoa powder

2¼ cups maple syrup

1 cup coconut butter

Blend all of the filling ingredients in a blender until smooth. Taste the ganache to make sure it's not grainy. If it is, continue blending further until completely smooth. Pour into the chilled tart crust. Lightly lift and drop the pan onto the counter to release any air bubbles. Place in the refrigerator to chill and set at least 3 hours.

For the vanilla cream:

1 cup raw cashews,
    soaked 4 hours or more

1 cup coconut meat

½ cup filtered water

½ cup agave nectar

½ cup coconut butter

2 tablespoons vanilla extract

Seeds of ½ vanilla bean (or 1 additional
    teaspoon vanilla extract)

¼ teaspoon salt

In a Vita-Mix or high-speed blender, blend all the vanilla cream ingredients until completely smooth. Transfer to a separate container and refrigerate to chill and set, 2 hours or more. This will make a firm, scoopable cream. For a slightly softer cream, use half the amount of coconut butter.

For serving:

1 Use a chef's knife to cut the tart in half. It helps to run the knife under hot water and then dry it with a towel between cuts in order to cut more smoothly. Cut each half in half again and each quarter into 3 pieces for 12 evenly sized slices.

2 Top each slice with a spoonful of the vanilla cream.

Cutting Out Coffee

It might be hard to picture beginning a morning or ending an evening meal without coffee. As a beverage, it really isn't that old: coffee was only first embraced in the thirteenth century by somnolent Arab monks who couldn't keep their minds on their prayers. From there, it was introduced to Europeans in the seventeenth century. Despite its common acceptance in our lives, coffee—and the caffeine it contains—might just be one of the biggest threats to our continued good health, both physical and mental.

Stephen Cherniske, in his seminal book *Caffeine Blues*, calls caffeine a "biological poison used by plants as a pesticide," noting that "caffeine gives leaves and seeds a bitter taste, which discourages their consumption by insects and animals. If predators insist on eating a caffeine-containing plant, the caffeine can cause central nervous system disruptions and even lethal side effects. Most pests soon learn to leave the plant alone." (This is why, incidentally, it's dangerous for your pets to eat commercial chocolate, which can contain large amounts of caffeine.)

Unfortunately, humans are the most persistent of pests, and we've found ways to make irresistibly palatable what is essentially a psychoactive drug that impairs us; the so-called "stimulating" effect of caffeine is merely your body stepping up the system to flush the poison out as quickly as possible. In fact, coffee beans were first employed as a drug to "detoxify" the sick. Caffeine has a similar chemical make-up to morphine, nicotine, and cocaine, to which very few of us with non-bling celeb status would be proud or solvent enough to admit an addiction. But it's not uncommon for us to claim that we can't function without our coffee.

Aside from being addictive, coffee is damaging to the liver, which has to detoxify the caffeine in it. Decaffeinated coffee is not an a-okay replacement. Decaf also contains a variety of damaging chemicals, including the same cancer-causing agents found in barbecued foods. And the decaffeinating process itself often uses chemicals.

Still, if the necessary organs can process moderate amounts of caffeine and related substances, why should we go cold turkey on coffee? Perhaps because daily doses of caffeine have been implicated in the following: gastrointestinal disease, sleep disorders, malnutrition (it drains the kidneys of the ability to hold onto calcium, magnesium, potassium, and zinc), headaches and depression. Plus every cup of coffee is a glass of body-refreshing water (one of the most important elements of a raw diet) you *didn't* drink.

Pineapple Carpaccio

with star anise syrup
and coconut ice cream

SERVES 6

Somehow, when pineapple flesh is sliced this thinly and then pressed, it becomes more delicate yet the flavor seems more intense. The star anise adds another layer of sweetness and spice. We keep pineapple sage plants in our garden at the restaurant and snip a few branches before service each night. Keep your herbs in cold water so they don't wilt if you will not be using them right away. Lemon basil, regular basil, or mint are all great substitutes for the pineapple sage.

> I made six quarts of this coconut ice cream and served it with chocolate cookies to all our restaurant staff during our first orientation meeting. I wanted them to see straightaway how yummy raw food can be. —SM

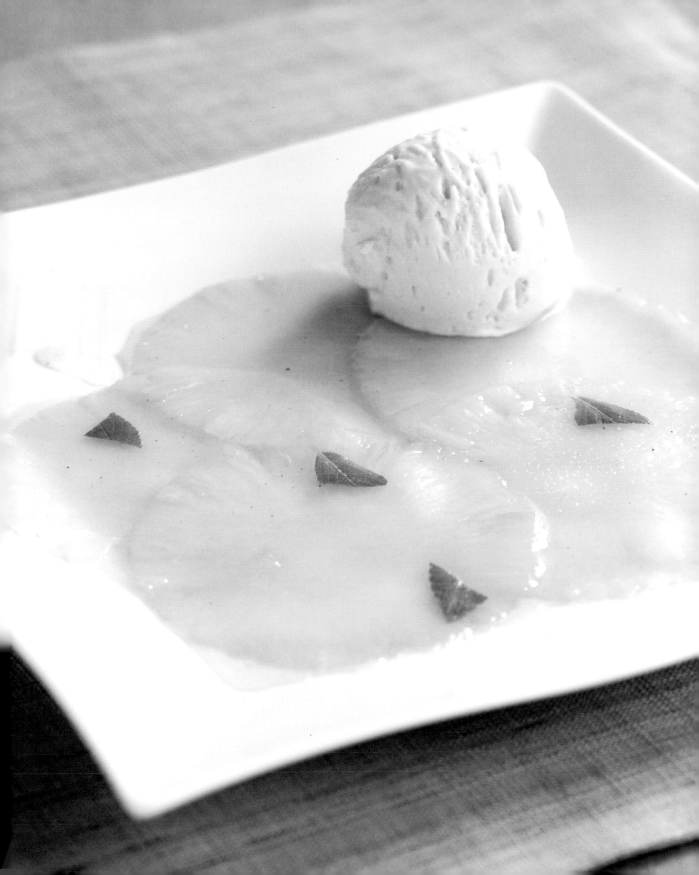

For the coconut ice cream:

1¹/₂ cups coconut meat
1¹/₂ cups coconut water
¹/₄ cup agave nectar
3 tablespoons coconut butter
¹/₂ teaspoon lemon or lime juice
Seeds from ¹/₂ vanilla bean (or 1 teaspoon vanilla extract)
3 packets stevia
¹/₄ teaspoon sea salt

In a Vita-Mix or high-speed blender, puree all ingredients until smooth. Chill completely in the refrigerator and then process in an ice cream maker according to the manufacturer's directions.

For the pineapple carpaccio:

1 ripe pineapple, top, bottom, and outer peel cut away
¹/₂ cup agave nectar
¹/₂ teaspoon ground star anise
1 small handful pineapple sage leaves or sliced or torn lemon basil or regular basil (optional)

1 At the restaurant, we slice the pineapple with a heavy duty slicer. At home, it's easiest to cut the pineapple in half lengthwise and then either use a Japanese mandoline or a sharp knife to get very thin slices, ¹/₄ to ¹/₆ inch thick.

2 Set out one of the plates on which you plan to serve the dessert. Cover it with a sheet of plastic wrap, leaving plenty of overhang on both sides. Arrange the pineapple slices, overlapping, to cover the plate. Lay another piece of plastic wrap over the pineapple, pressing down to smooth it. Slide the pineapple onto a flat surface and, using your palm, press down uniformly to flatten it a bit. Fold up the sides of the plastic wrap to make a neat package. Repeat with the remaining pineapple. Stack the pineapple packages and lay them flat in the freezer for 30 minutes or more, until ready to serve.

3 In a small bowl, stir together the agave nectar and star anise.

4 To serve, remove the pineapple packages from the freezer. Lay each one flat and run your hands over them to help them thaw a bit. Peel off the top layer of plastic and invert onto a serving plate. Carefully peel back the remaining plastic. Spoon a bit of the star anise syrup over the pineapple. Place a scoop of coconut ice cream in the corner and garnish with the pineapple sage, if using, and serve immediately.

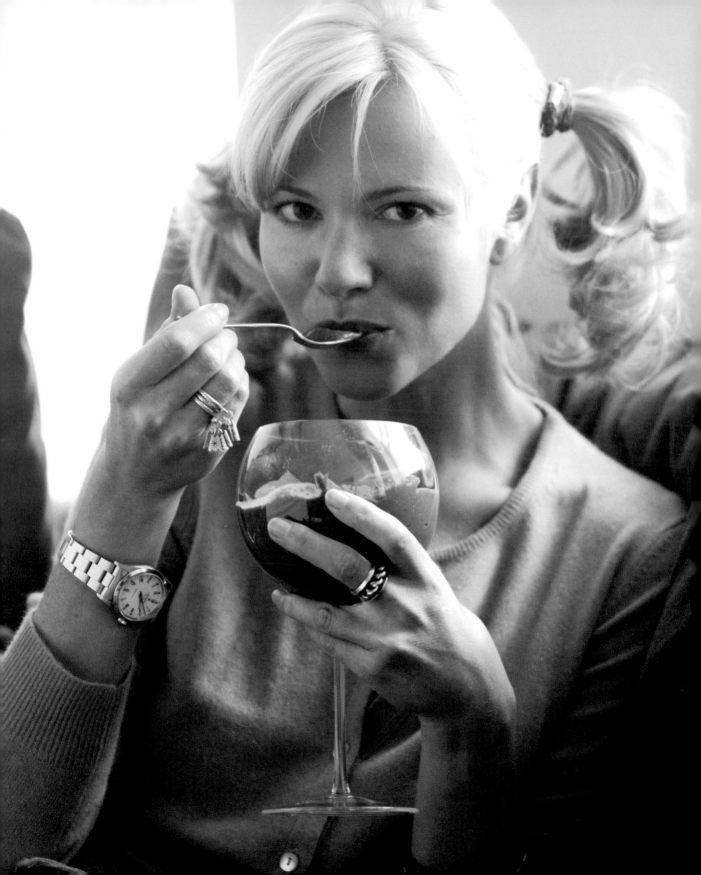

Chocolate Pudding

This recipe is so simple and easy—it takes only a few minutes (not including the coconut whacking). You can substitute carob for the cocoa, as regular cocoa powder is usually ground from roasted cacao beans and therefore not really raw. If you are using a Vita-Mix, you can add a bit of raw cacao beans to the blender in place of some of the cocoa powder, for a bit more intense flavor.

> **Matthew made this one night at home when he felt like something creamy with chocolate, and it's been extremely popular at our take-out since we opened. It's creamy and rich tasting—people are always shocked that there is no dairy in it.** —SM

2 cups coconut meat
³/₄ cup coconut water, at room temperature (or more, if needed to thin)
¹/₂ cup maple syrup
¹/₃ cup agave nectar
¹/₂ cup cocoa powder
2 tablespoons vanilla extract
¹/₄ teaspoon sea salt

In a Vita-Mix or high-speed blender, puree all the ingredients until completely smooth, stopping to scrape the sides as necessary. Transfer to bowls and chill for a firmer pudding, or eat it straightaway. Try this with raspberries and fresh mint, or chopped nuts.

Sour Cherry Tart
with almond cream

MAKES ABOUT TEN 4 ½-INCH TARTS OR TWENTY 3-INCH TARTS

This can also be made with blueberries or raspberries, and is especially pretty with the tiny wild Maine blueberries or wild-from-anywhere raspberries. It could be topped with any fruit, really, as long as it's not a watery fruit that will make the cream underneath it runny. The recipe calls for both coarse and fine almond flour. Of course, you can just grind the almonds and use 3 cups total, rather than separating between the coarse and fine crumbs. However, to make a slightly more refined crust, you may want to sift through the nut crumbs to remove any larger pieces—either way it will taste the same.

We use cashews to make the almond cream—which seems odd, but we found that almonds are a bit too grainy and cashews make a much smoother cream. Organic almond extract provides the almond flavor that goes so well with cherries, but you can leave it out or add more vanilla bean if you prefer.

> **Sarma's mother dropped off a huge box of fresh sour cherries from her farm in New Hampshire, and Debbie made this tart. Keeping the cherries warm in the dehydrator until just before you serve it is a nice touch.** —MK

For the cherry topping:

6 cups sour cherries, stemmed and pitted
½ cup agave nectar
2 teaspoons vanilla extract

In a medium bowl, toss the cherries with the agave nectar and the vanilla. Transfer to Teflex-lined dehydrator trays and dehydrate at 115°F for 3 to 4 hours, or until they have softened and are warmed through.

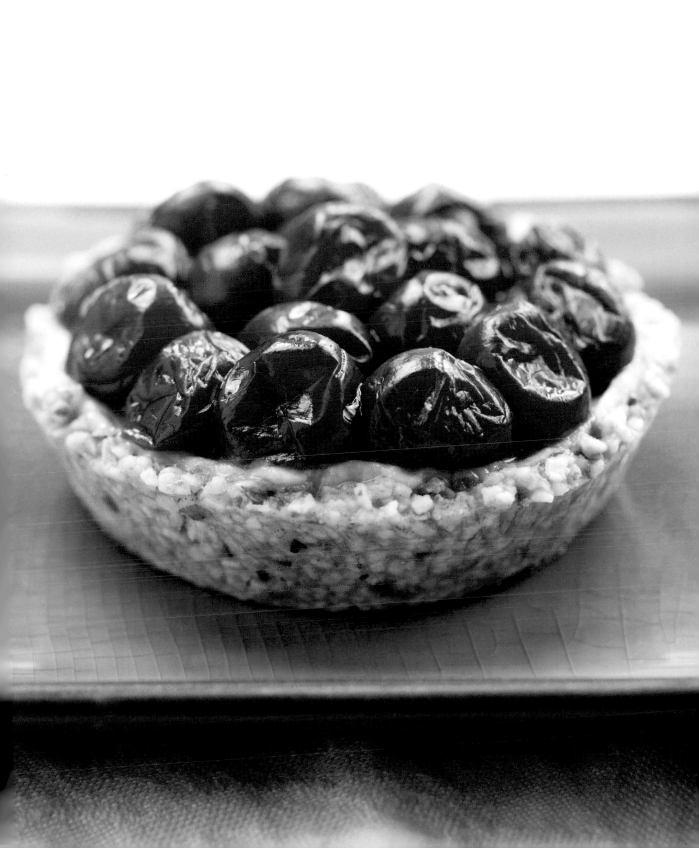

For the tart crusts:

1½ cups coarse almond flour (page 230)
1½ cups fine almond flour (page 230)
3 tablespoons date paste

¾ cup maple syrup powder
¾ cup coconut butter
Large pinch of sea salt

In a medium bowl, mix together all the crust ingredients until very thoroughly combined. Line individual tart shells with squares of plastic wrap. Divide the dough between the shells and press evenly into the sides and bottom, to create an even thickness throughout. Refrigerate until firm, about 1 hour or more, and keep refrigerated until ready to fill.

For the almond cream:

1 cup raw cashews,
    soaked 2 hours or more
1 cup coconut meat
⅔ cup agave nectar
¼ to ½ cup filtered water,
    at room temperature

6 tablespoons coconut butter
1 tablespoon plus 1 teaspoon
    pure almond extract
Seeds from ½ vanilla bean,
    or 2 teaspoons vanilla extract
Pinch of sea salt

1 In a Vita-Mix or high-speed blender, puree all the cream ingredients until completely smooth, stopping to scrape the sides as necessary. Use the tamper that comes with the Vita-Mix, if you have it, to push the mix down into the blades for easier blending. Add more coconut water to thin, but avoid adding too much or the cream will not stay as firm in the tart shells.

2 Fill each tart crust with the cream, creating a flat surface at the top. Cover and return to the refrigerator to chill and set, about 2 hours or more.

For the serving:

Remove the tarts from the refrigerator and use the overhanging edges of the plastic wrap to carefully pull the tarts from the shells (or push from the bottom if using shells with removable bottoms). Arrange the warm cherries on top of each and serve.

Lime Mousse Tart
with coconut macadamia crust

MAKES 4 SMALL TARTS

The mousse can be served in bowls on its own if you don't feel like making the crusts. Nobody ever guesses that the main ingredient in this mousse is avocado. The coconut butter can be omitted from the mousse—it's in the recipe to provide stiffness (as coconut butter becomes solid when chilled) but it is not critical. This recipe uses a lot of stevia; using too much of a liquid sweetener will make the mousse runny. You can always substitute a bit of maple or date sugar if you like, but it will slightly alter the color of the mousse.

> **If someone threw one of these pies in your face, it would be like an avocado mask.** —SM

For the tart crust:

2 cups raw macadamia nuts
1 cup shredded, unsweetened dry coconut
1 tablespoon lime zest
2 tablespoons lime juice
Seeds from ½ vanilla bean, or 2 teaspoons vanilla extract
1 teaspoon sea salt
4 packets stevia
2 tablespoons agave nectar
1 tablespoon macadamia oil, or other nut oil

1 Place the nuts and the processor bowl in the freezer to chill for a few minutes. Once chilled, place all of the ingredients except the oil in the processor bowl and pulse until well combined, but still a bit chunky. Be careful not to overprocess or the nuts will become oily.

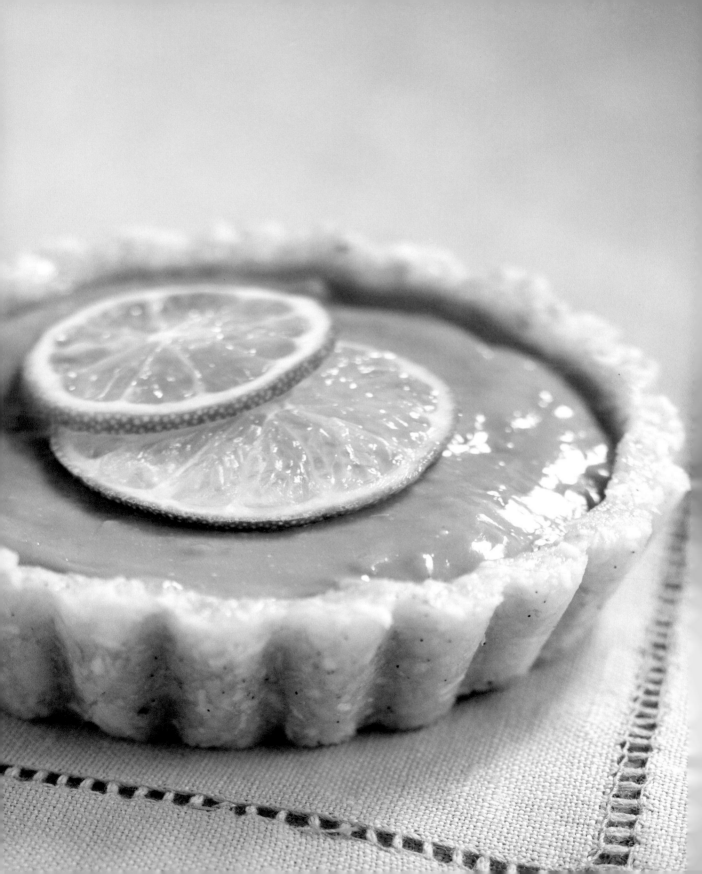

2 Lightly oil four 4-inch tart shells with removable bottoms with the macadamia oil. If using tart shells without removable bottoms, line the pans with overhanging plastic wrap, and skip oiling them. Divide the dough into four parts and press into the tart shells. When the shells are filled, wrap in plastic and place in the freezer to chill until firm.

For the lime mousse:

5 ripe avocados, peeled and pitted
$^1/_2$ cup lime juice
$^1/_4$ cup packed lime zest (from 6 to 8 limes)
$^1/_4$ cup agave nectar
2 tablespoons coconut butter
Seeds from $^1/_2$ vanilla bean, or 2 teaspoons vanilla extract
$^1/_2$ teaspoon sea salt
10 packets stevia (or to taste)

1 In the bowl of a food processor, process all the mousse ingredients except the stevia until smooth. Add stevia to taste and process.

2 Use the overhanging edges of the plastic wrap to carefully pull the tarts from the shells (or push from the bottom if using shells with removable bottoms). Fill the tart shells with the mousse, cover with wax paper, parchment, or plastic wrap and chill in the refrigerator or freezer. Do not leave the filled tarts uncovered for too long or the surface may discolor a bit—it's best to cover the surface directly with the wax paper or parchment, which will peel off easily once chilled. If you freeze the tarts, allow them to thaw gently for at least 15 minutes before serving.

ALTERNATE PREPARATION: In the restaurant we use ring molds. Press the crust dough onto parchment about $^1/_3$-inch thick, press the molds into it to cut out rounds and then fill the rings with mousse and chill. To unmold, soak a clean kitchen towel in hot water and hold it around the molds for a bit—the rings should then easily slide off.

Pumpkin Tart

with candied pumpkin seeds

This recipe makes enough crust for about 10 tarts if you are using 4½-inch shells. At the restaurant we use 3-inch shells, which are a nice size for a small dessert. Smooth-sided tart shells work best for this recipe, but any kind will do. If you try making a large tart, the crust should be a bit thicker to withstand the pressure of removing it from the shell or using a tart ring would work well too. As with the sour cherry tart, the recipe calls for both coarse and fine almond flour. Again, you can just grind the almonds and use 3 cups total, rather than separating between the coarse and fine crumbs. However, to make a slightly more refined crust, you may want to sift through the nut crumbs to remove any larger pieces—either way it will taste the same.

Try also serving it with the Vanilla Cream (page 232) spiced with a generous pinch of ground ginger.

> **This dessert was created for our fall menu by Emily Cavelier and we think it's far better than traditional pumpkin pie (which is generally made with gelatinous canned and pasteurized pumpkin). This version tastes fresher and more vibrant—and if you don't tell, no one will ever guess that there's not any actual pumpkin in it.** —MK

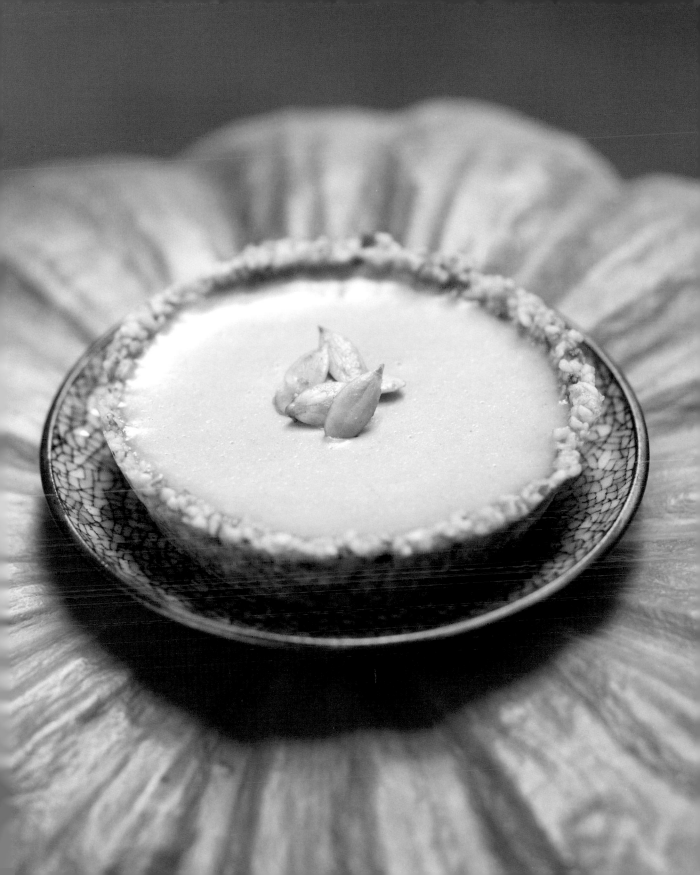

For the tart crusts:

1½ cups coarse almond flour (page 230)
1½ cups fine almond flour (page 230)
3 tablespoons date paste

¾ cup maple syrup powder
¾ cup coconut butter
Large pinch of sea salt

In a medium bowl, mix together all the ingredients until very thoroughly combined. Line ten 4½-inch or twenty 3-inch tart shells with squares of plastic wrap. Divide the dough between the shells and press evenly into the sides and bottom, to create an even thickness throughout. Refrigerate until firm, about 1 hour or more, and keep refrigerated until ready to fill.

For the filling:

1 cup raw cashews, soaked 4 hours or more
1 cup coconut meat
2 cups carrot juice
¾ cup agave nectar
¾ cup coconut butter
⅓ cup date paste

1 tablespoon vanilla extract
1 tablespoon ground cinnamon
2 teaspoons ground ginger
½ teaspoon ground nutmeg
¼ teaspoon ground cloves
¾ teaspoon sea salt

In a Vita-Mix or high-speed blender, blend all the filling ingredients until completely smooth. Fill the tart shells while the filling is still at room temperature. Place the tart shells in the refrigerator to set, about 1 hour or more. You may have extra filling, in which case simply chill it and eat it like pudding!

For serving:

1 cup Candied Pumpkin Seeds (page 288)

Carefully release the tarts from the shells and discard the plastic. Top each tart with a few spiced candied pumpkin seeds. If not serving immediately, store in the refrigerator. Ideally, let the tarts sit at room temperature for 15 to 20 minutes before serving, so they are not too cold.

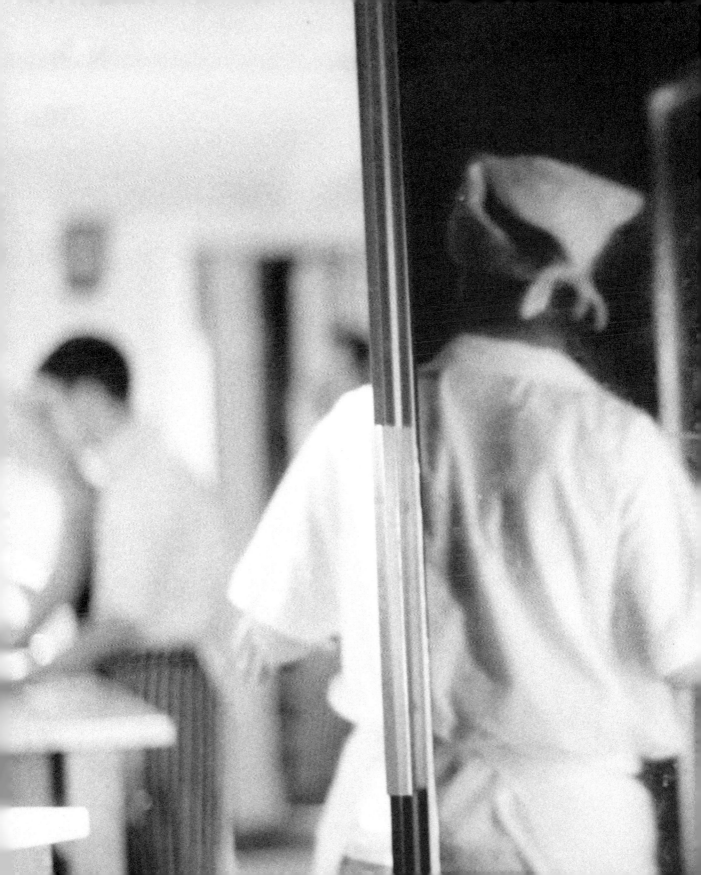

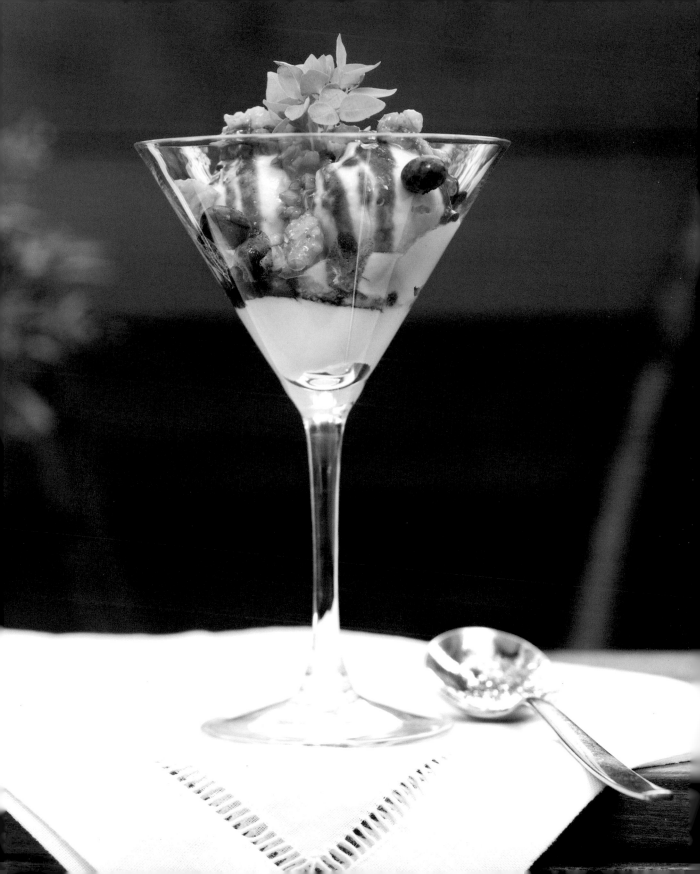

Lavender Ice Cream and Blueberry Sundae

SERVES 4 TO 6

Lavender is not just for tea or a bubble bath—though it's nice in both! You can find it fresh at greenmarkets. If not, try another herb, such as chamomile, and serve it with blackberries, or mint paired with little wild strawberries. Blueberries are full of pectin that gels up when it sits, so you may need to stir and/or shake the sauce before serving.

> " Sometimes a dessert should just be rich and creamy without any fussy presentations or delicate pastry. Although the flavors in this sundae are sophisticated and unique, it is ultimately a simple, satisfying final course. " —MK

For the ice cream:

2 cups raw cashews, soaked 4 hours or more
2 cups coconut meat
1 cup filtered water
1 cup agave nectar
$1/2$ cup coconut butter
2 tablespoons edible organic lavender flowers
2 teaspoons vanilla extract
$1/2$ teaspoon sea salt

In a Vita-Mix or high-speed blender, blend all the ice cream ingredients until completely smooth. Chill thoroughly in the refrigerator and then process in an ice cream maker according to the manufacturer's instructions.

For the blueberry sauce:

2 cups blueberries
$1/3$ cup agave nectar

1 Place the blueberries on a dehydrator tray and dehydrate at 115°F for 4 to 6 hours, or until they begin to look a bit shrunken. This will concentrate the flavors a bit, but is not a necessary step if you do not have the time.

2 Place 1 $1/2$ cups of the blueberries in a blender with the agave nectar and puree until smooth. Transfer to a small bowl and stir in the remaining $1/2$ cup blueberries.

For serving:

$1/2$ cup Candied Walnuts (page 294)
Lemon basil leaves, for garnish (or use sprigs of lavender or other herbs)

Spoon the ice cream into serving dishes, top with blueberry sauce and walnuts, and garnish with herbs.

Vanilla Ice Cream

We use both vanilla extract and vanilla beans because the beans are so expensive, but if you want, by all means, use all beans and skip the extract.

> This ice cream is a great base for all kinds of flavor variations. We've had so many on our dessert menu since we opened. Add a few fresh peppermint leaves to the blender and then stir in raw cacao nibs to make mint chocolate chip. Or stir in Maple Sugared Slivered Almonds (page 294) for our favorite almond brittle ice cream. —MK

2 cups raw cashews, soaked 4 hours or more
2 cups coconut meat
1 cup filtered water
1 cup agave nectar
$^1/_4$ cup coconut butter
2 tablespoons vanilla extract
Seeds of $^1/_2$ vanilla bean, or 2 additional teaspoons vanilla extract
$^1/_2$ teaspoon sea salt

In a Vita-Mix or high-speed blender, blend all the ingredients until completely smooth. Chill thoroughly in the refrigerator and then process in an ice cream maker according to the manufacturer's instructions.

Concord Grape Sorbet

Concord grapes are amazing, full of so much flavor and sweetness. They are available at our greenmarket from late August through October, where you can smell them from a distance.

SERVES 6 TO 8

> " I love this sorbet, and its intense purple color. Eat it with the Almond Butter Cookies (page 260) and you get a PB&J effect. " —SM

4 cups concord grapes
1 cup agave nectar
1 cup filtered water

In a Vita-Mix or high-speed blender, blend the grapes, agave nectar, and water until smooth. Pass through a fine-mesh strainer, discarding the solids. Chill thoroughly in the refrigerator and then process in an ice cream maker according to the manufacturer's instructions.

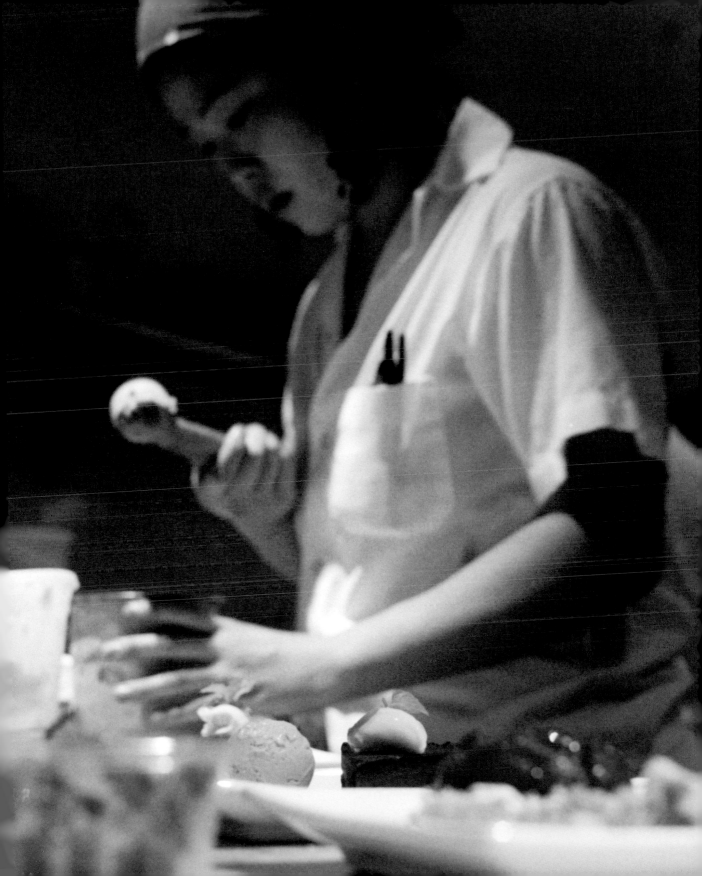

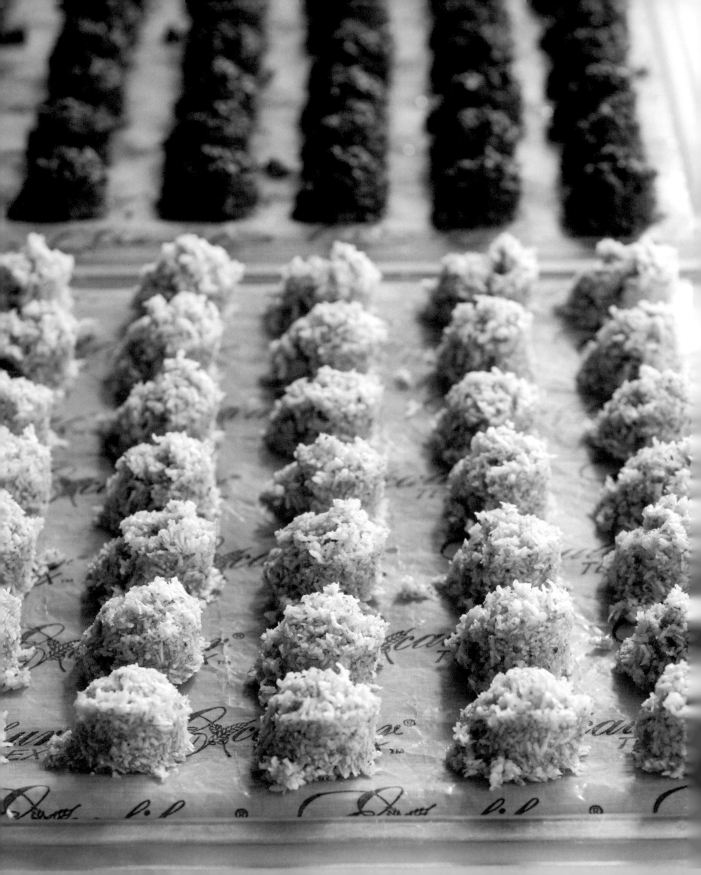

Macaroons
Chocolate or Blonde

MAKES 24 TO 36 MACAROONS

These are the bestseller, by far, in our take-out store. As always, you can use carob in place of cocoa powder. We started with the chocolate version and then added the blonde variety—both are so good, we can never decide which we like better.

> **Sarma and I used to make macaroons at home, but then our pastry chef, Emily, took them to the next level at the restaurant and created the vanilla version as well.** —MK

3 cups dried, unsweetened coconut flakes
1¹/₂ cups cocoa powder
1 cup maple syrup

¹/₃ cup coconut butter
1 tablespoon vanilla extract
¹/₂ teaspoon sea salt

1 In a large bowl, combine all the ingredients and stir well to combine. You can also use a standing mixer with the paddle attachment.

2 Using a small ice cream scoop, your hands, or a big tablespoon, spoon rounds of the dough onto dehydrator screens. If you are using your hands, it helps to refrigerate the mix a bit prior to forming the macaroons. Dehydrate at 115°F for 12 to 24 hours, or until crisp on the outside and nice and chewy on the inside.

FOR BLONDE MACAROONS: Replace the cocoa powder in the recipe above with an equal amount of fine almond flour (see page 230).

Cherry Pistachio Biscotti

MAKES 18 TO 24 BISCOTTI

Try adding raw cacao nibs to these, or chopped dried apricot in place of the cherries. They are great with tea, and even better dipped in a nice glass of Vin Santo—the traditional way to eat biscotti.

> While I used to love the taste of biscotti filled with refined white sugar and flour, this variation has more complex flavor and substance. And they actually feed your body. —MK

6 cups coarse almond flour (page 230)
6 tablespoons date paste
1 cup dried cherries, coarsely chopped
³/₄ cup raw pistachios
1 cup plus 2 tablespoons maple or date sugar
³/₄ teaspoon sea salt

1 In a large bowl, blend all the ingredients by hand until thoroughly combined. Divide the dough in half and shape directly on Teflex sheets into two long rectangles, slightly mounded in the center. Slide the Teflex sheets onto dehydrator screens and dehydrate at 115°F for 2 to 3 hours, or until the outsides feel dry.

2 Remove the dough from the dehydrator and cut into bars about ³/₄ inch wide. Place them directly onto the dehydrator screens and dehydrate further for 12 hours or more, until slightly crisp.

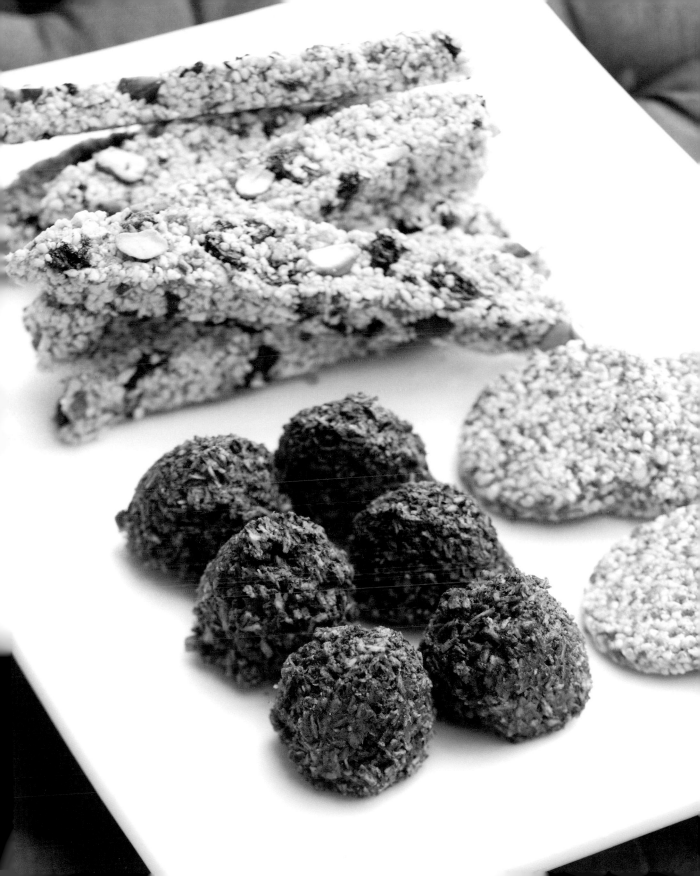

Almond Butter Cookies

> " These are crunchy and good for you. And if you really love
> almonds, you can eat them with almond milk. " —SM

4 cups coarse almond flour (page 230)

1 cup almond butter

3 tablespoons agave nectar

$^1/_2$ cup raw honey or date paste

2 teaspoons vanilla extract

2 teaspoons sea salt

2 packets stevia (optional)

1 In a large bowl, combine all the ingredients, stirring well. You can also use a standing mixer with the paddle attachment.

2 Transfer the dough onto a sheet of parchment or wax paper, or a Teflex sheet. Cover with another sheet of parchment, wax paper, or Teflex. With a rolling pin, roll out the dough into an even thickness, $^1/_4$ to $^1/_2$ inch thick. You may need to do this in two batches. Remove the top layer of paper or the Teflex and use a circular cutter to cut out cookies, or cut into any shape. With a flat spatula, carefully transfer the cookies to dehydrator screens. Like any cookie dough, scraps can be rerolled and recut until you use it all up.

3 Dehydrate the cookies at 115°F for 12 to 24 hours, or until crisp. Store in a covered container in the refrigerator for up to a week.

Chewy Chocolate Freezer Fudge

MAKES ABOUT 64 1" SQUARE PIECES (ABOUT ¾" THICK)

We call this "freezer fudge" because it is incredibly chewy when chilled. If you keep it out for too long it will melt.

> **I made these one night when I was procrastinating writing recipes, wandering away from the computer in search of something yummy to eat. Since then, Matthew and I have both been making them on a regular basis. I love using coarse salt, so you can taste the individual grains. We make them with raw carob powder (which gives it a caramel flavor) more often than with cocoa powder.** —SM

2 cups almond butter (one 16-ounce jar)
¼ cup cocoa powder, or raw carob powder, sifted to remove any lumps

½ cup plus 2 tablespoons maple syrup
1 heaping tablespoon coconut butter
2 teaspoons vanilla extract
1 teaspoon coarse sea salt

1 In a large bowl, combine all the ingredients, stirring well. You can also use a standing mixer with the paddle attachment, but it's more fun to do by hand.

2 Spoon the mixture into little candy molds, flatten with a spoon, and cover with parchment or wax paper. Or line a square baking pan with parchment or plastic. Place the fudge into the pan and cover the surface with parchment or wax paper, pressing down evenly to flatten. Place in the freezer to chill. If using the pan, remove from the freezer after an hour or so, flip it out of the pan onto a flat surface and cut into squares or rectangles. These should be stored, covered, in the freezer (otherwise they will get too soft and mushy) where they would keep quite well for a long time if they didn't always get eaten so fast.

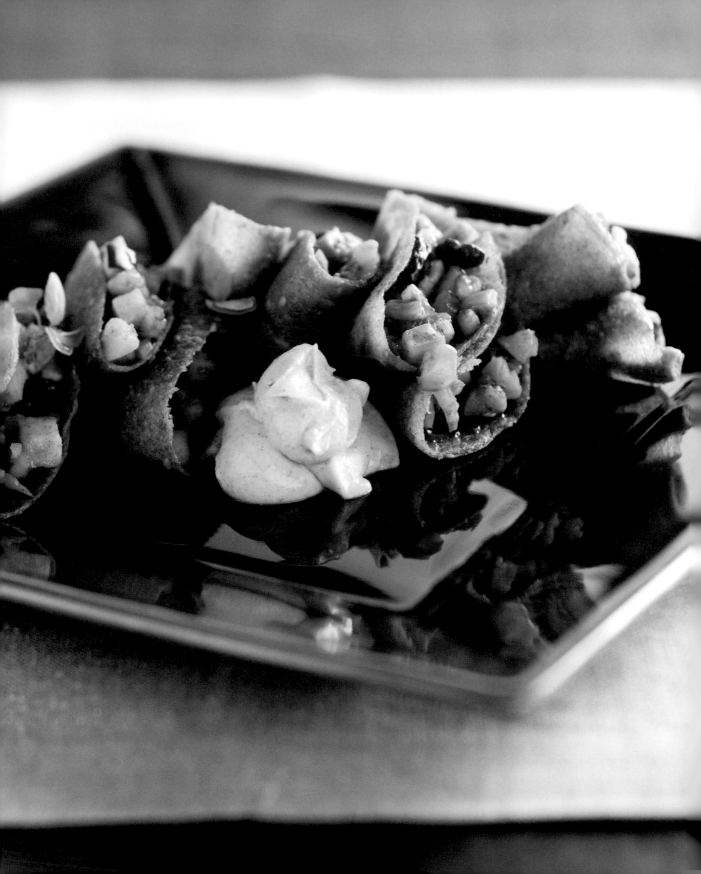

BREAKFAST AND BRUNCH

Raw food tenets recommend that you eat lightly in the morning; your body has been resting all night and it's something of an assault to bombard your system with food and force it to begin the work of digestion first thing.

That said, if you are very athletic or trying to add weight, a more substantial meal may be in order. Just give yourself enough time to get acclimated after you wake up.

Shakes and juices are ideal breakfasts. But if you have time or company on hand, you will want to explore some more intriguing dishes. In general, these recipes are *not* quick to prepare. In their favor, however, some are easily made ahead in large batches, and will last a long time if you store them in the fridge. For anyone who loves their weekend relaxation and the long, laid-back get-togethers it often entails, these recipes are ideal for lingering over, and pair magically with organic mimosas.

Apple Crepes

with apple walnut filling
and cinnamon maple cream

SERVES 4

You can peel the apple for the crepes but it's not necessary. In fact, the peel is where most of the nutrients are, so we like to keep it on whenever possible (although if for some reason you are not using organic apples, we always recommend peeling).

> " Our two current chefs, Glory Mongin and Amanda Cohen, developed this dish for our brunch menu. It's perfect for fall, and in the summertime instead of apples, you can substitute nectarines in the crepes and any stone fruits or berries in the filling, and maybe almonds for the walnuts. Try flavoring the crepes and cream with ginger instead of maple and cinnamon. " —SM

For the crepes:

3 cups coconut meat
1¹/₂ cup chopped apple
¹/₂ to 1 cup filtered water
1 cup golden flaxseed, finely ground (about 1¹/₃ cup ground)
3 tablespoons agave nectar
2 teaspoons ground cinnamon
1 teaspoon sea salt

1 In a Vita-Mix or high-speed blender, blend the coconut meat with the apple, adding the water ¹/₄ cup at a time as needed to make it smooth. You may need to use the tamper (the large black baton-like thing that comes with your Vita-Mix) to push the apple and coconut into the blades. The mixture should be thick, like a custard.

2 Transfer the coconut mixture to a large mixing bowl and add the ground flax, agave, cinnamon, and salt. Mix it very thoroughly with a spatula or large spoon.

3 Divide the batter between three 14-inch Teflex-lined dehydrator trays. Using an offset spatula, spread to about ¹/₆-inch thick. Dehydrate at 115°F for 6 to 8 hours or overnight. Flip them over and peel away the Teflex. Continue dehydrating on the screens only for another hour or two, until the underside is just dry and the crepes are still pliable.

4 Slide the crepes onto a flat cutting surface. Using a circle cutter (or you can trace around a small plate with a sharp knife), cut circles approximately 4 inches in diameter.

For the apple walnut filling:

4 cups cubed apple (skins on, about ¼-inch cubes), from about 4 apples
¾ cup coarsely chopped walnuts
¼ cup raisins
3 tablespoons maple syrup
3 tablespoons lemon juice (more or less depending on sweetness of apples)
½ teaspoon grated lemon zest
½ teaspoon ground cinnamon
¼ teaspoon sea salt

Toss all the filling ingredients in a bowl. Spread on a Teflex-lined dehydrator tray and dehydrate at 115°F for 1 to 2 hours, just to soften the apples a bit.

For the maple cream:

½ cup cashews, soaked 2 hours or more
½ cup coconut meat
½ cup maple syrup
2 tablespoons coconut butter
¼ cup filtered water
2 teaspoons vanilla extract
¼ teaspoon ground cinnamon
¼ teaspoon sea salt

In a Vita-Mix or high-speed blender, blend all the maple cream ingredients thoroughly. Transfer to a bowl and refrigerate if not using right away.

For the assembly:

Maple syrup
Fresh mint for garnish (optional)

Fill each of the crepes with the apple walnut filling and fold. Serve with the maple cream, drizzle with maple syrup, and garnish with fresh mint, if desired.

Spiced Oatmeal with Dried Fruits

SERVES 4 TO 6

While this recipe requires quite a long soaking time—five days!—the rest is easy. You can cut down the soaking time by using warm water, or eat it sooner if you don't mind a little more coarseness to your oatmeal. Oats are quite high in protein, fiber, B vitamins, calcium, iron, and folic acid. If you're a pregnant raw foodist, this is the breakfast of future champions.

> **Sarma had a recipe for oatmeal cookies that she gave to our pastry department to test, and Elena Baletta, who works with us, made this great oatmeal for our brunch menu. It's really nice warmed in the dehydrator, or with chopped fresh apple or sliced banana and nut milk.** —MK

3 cups oat groats, soaked 5 days
1 cup maple syrup
2 cups golden raisins
1 tablespoon ground cinnamon
$^1/_2$ teaspoon sea salt
2 cups dark raisins

1 Soak the oatmeal in water for 5 days, changing the water and briefly rinsing the oats at least once per day.

2 Drain all of the excess water from the oats. In a food processor, pulse together the oats, syrup, golden raisins, cinnamon, and salt until the oats are broken down and the mix is an oatmeal-like consistency—as smooth or chunky as you prefer. Transfer to a bowl and fold in the dark raisins.

Cranberry Maple Granola

MAKES ABOUT 10 CUPS

This granola, or *grawnola*, as we call it at the take-out store, is hearty and crunchy. It's a really good snack to have around or to take with you when traveling, although we like it best as a cereal with berries and sweet Brazil nut milk. You can easily vary the recipe, substituting chopped dried apples for the cranberries and ginger powder for the orange zest.

> " Storing this granola in the refrigerator helps it to stay crunchy and it keeps really well for quite a long time. Although I'm not exactly sure how I would know that since it always gets eaten within a few days. " —MK

1 apple, cored and chopped
1 1/2 cups date paste
1/3 cup maple syrup
2 tablespoons lemon juice
2 tablespoons orange zest
1 tablespoon vanilla extract
1 teaspoon ground cinnamon
2 teaspoons sea salt
1/2 cup sunflower seeds, soaked 2 hours or more
2 cups almonds, soaked 4 hours or more
3 cups pecans, soaked 2 hours or more
1 cup pumpkin seeds, soaked 2 hours or more
1 cup dried cranberries

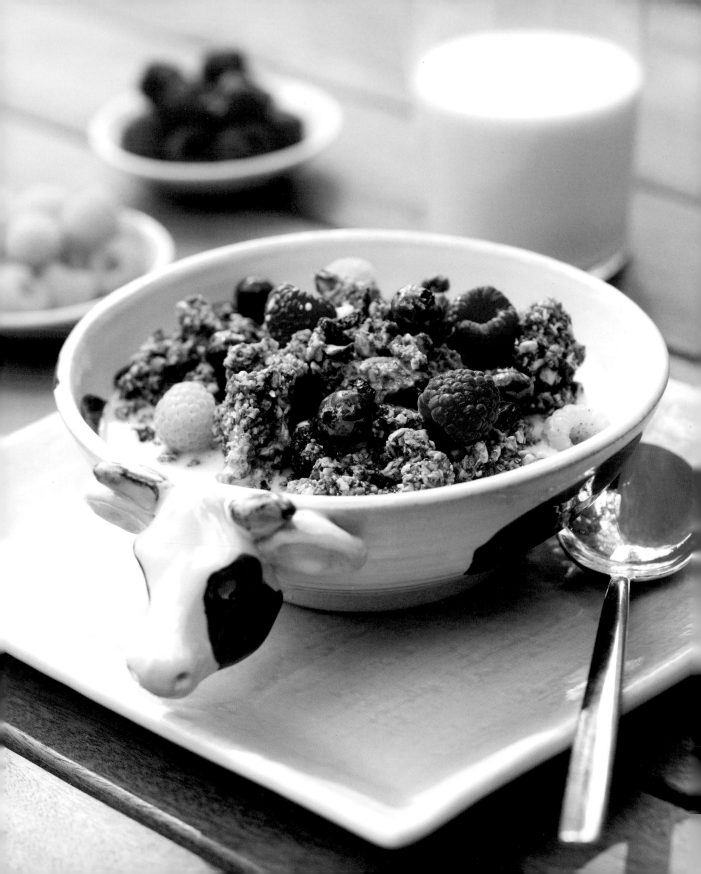

1 In a food processor, place the apple, date paste, maple syrup, lemon juice, orange zest, vanilla, cinnamon, salt, and 1/4 cup of the sunflower seeds and grind until completely smooth. Transfer the mixture to a large mixing bowl.

2 Add the remaining 1/4 cup sunflower seeds, the almonds, pecans, and pumpkin seeds to the food processor (you don't need to bother rinsing the bowl in between). Coarsely chop the nuts and seeds in a few quick pulses. Add them to the bowl with the apple mixture, add the cranberries and combine well.

3 Spread the granola on Teflex-lined dehydrator trays and dehydrate at 115°F for 6 to 8 hours. Flip the granola over onto the screens and peel away the Teflex. Continue dehydrating for another 8 to 12 hours, or until the granola is crunchy. Break into pieces and, once completely cooled, store in an airtight container. To maintain freshness longer, store the granola in the refrigerator for up to a few weeks.

Maple Cinnamon Buckwheat Crispies

& cocoa crispies

SERVES 4 TO 6

One of the things we missed a bit when we went raw was eating cereal. Our buckwheat version, served in a bowl with Brazil nut milk and berries or sliced banana, is better tasting and so much better for you than the processed kinds. Technically, buckwheat is not a grain but an edible fruit seed. Moreover, it's basic and easy to digest, as opposed to grains, which form acids and upset the pH balance of the body. Its compatibility to the digestive system is evident in the way it softens so quickly when you soak it; in 1 hour it goes completely soft, whereas grains can take hours or even days and still do not get that soft. Make sure to purchase whole, raw buckwheat groats, not the toasted kind known as *kashi*.

> **I made a lot of this our first summer eating raw in Maine. It's very quick and easy to make. And, not to sound like a TV commercial, but it stays really crispy in nut milk, too. Our stylist for the photo shoots, Bette, brought some home to her kids and they loved it!** —SM

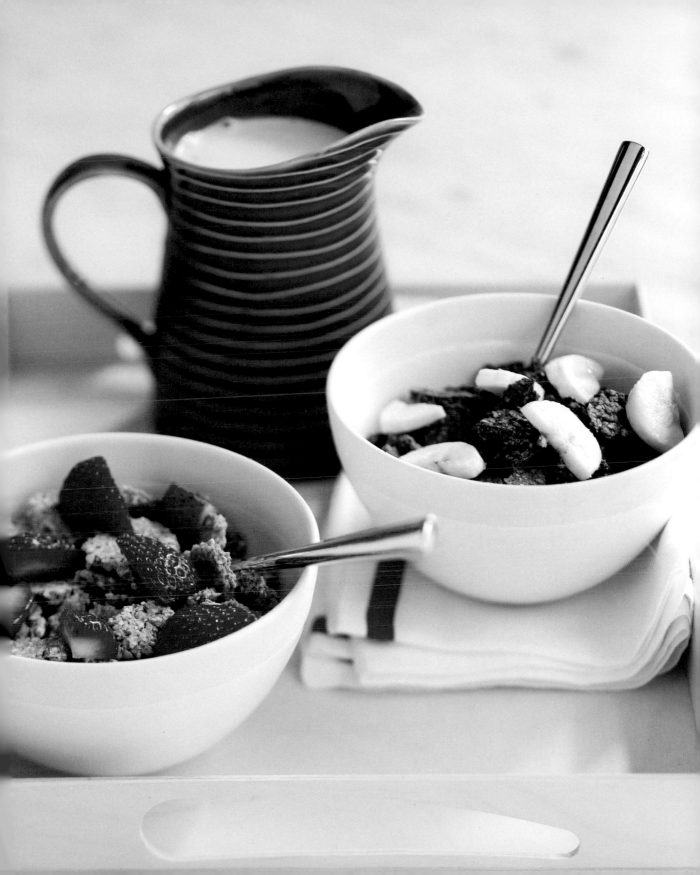

2 cups buckwheat groats, soaked for at least 1 hour (will yield about 3¹/₂ cups)
³/₄ cup maple syrup
1¹/₂ teaspoons vanilla extract
1 teaspoon ground cinnamon
2 packets stevia
2 teaspoons sea salt

1 Place the soaked buckwheat groats in a fine-mesh colander to drain. Rinse with water to get rid of extra starchiness.

2 Place in the bowl of a food processor and add the remaining ingredients. Pulse until very well combined but not thoroughly pureed. It should look somewhat like soupy oatmeal.

3 Divide between two Teflex-lined dehydrator trays and spread to about ¹/₈-inch thickness. Dehydrate at 115°F for 8 to 12 hours or until the top is dry to the touch and the Teflex peels away easily. The crispies should be quite brittle at this point, so it would be hard to flip it over all in one piece—the best way is to lift up pieces and flip them over individually. Continue dehydrating for an additional few hours, or until they are completely dry and crunchy. Break into pieces and store in an airtight container, or keep in the fridge to maintain maximum freshness, where they should last up to a few weeks.

COCOA CRISPIES Replace the cinnamon with 2 heaping tablespoons of organic cocoa powder or carob powder.

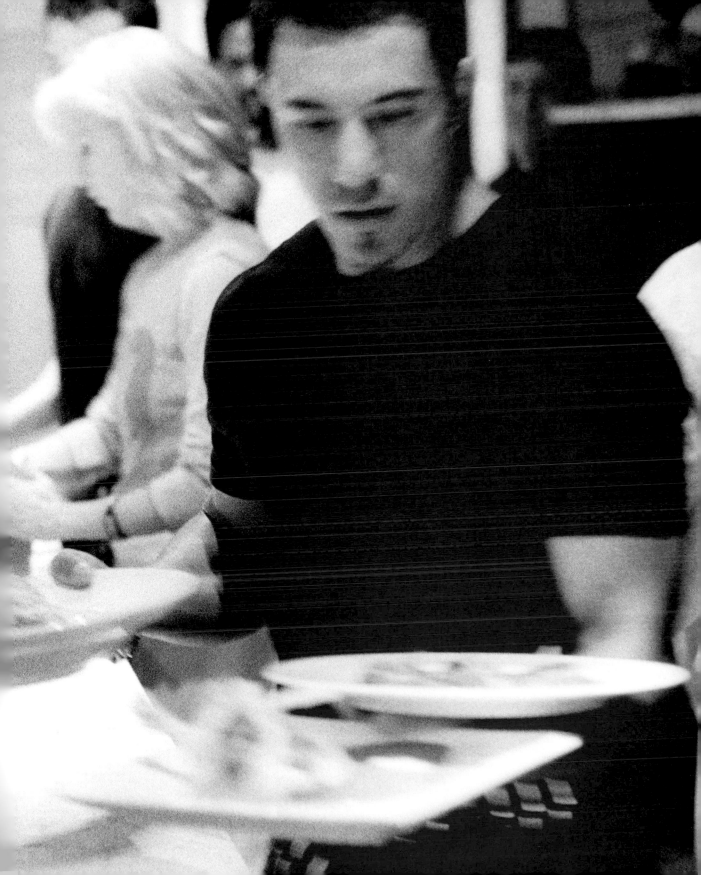

Crunchy Honey Nut Butter and Berry Jam Sandwich

MAKES 4 SANDWICHES

Raw almond butter on its own is a bit too runny to hold up in a sandwich. Mixing it with raw honey, which should always be solid rather than liquid at room temperature, will give it more body, not to mention a great taste. We always stir coarse sea salt into our almond butter every time we open a jar as well, as it usually comes unsalted. Dehydrating the strawberries to concentrate the flavors will also give them more substance for the jam. And dehydrating the bread makes it a bit more like toast. Because it is not baked at a high temperature, manna bread, is still somewhat wet and muffin-like on the inside. You can buy it frozen in any health food store. It's a very convenient snack to have on hand. There is some debate about whether or not it's truly raw, because we've yet been able to find out for sure if they keep it at less than 118°F—but in any case, it's the best sort of "bread" you could buy to eat, because they use fully sprouted organic grains and presumably keep it uncooked, so it's a big step in the right direction.

> **You can make all the components of this ahead of time and keep them refrigerated. Then, whether it's for a late morning breakfast or a snack any time of day, it's easy to put together. Just like those peanut butter and jelly sandwiches that I remember eating every day for lunch in school, but so much better!** —MK

8 slices Manna bread, preferably cinnamon date, cut into slices about $^1/_2$ inch thick (see Sources, page 364)

2 pints strawberries, trimmed and cut in pieces

2 tablespoons agave nectar

1 packet stevia or 3 tablespoons maple syrup powder (optional, see Sources, page 364)

1 cup raw almond butter

$^1/_2$ cup raw honey

$^1/_2$ teaspoon sea salt

1 Place the slices of bread on dehydrator trays and dehydrate at 115°F for 4 to 8 hours, or until a bit crispy on the outside. This is not necessary, but we like the recipe better when the bread is a bit more dry and toast-like.

2 Place the strawberries on Teflex-lined dehydrator trays and dehydrate at 115°F for 6 to 8 hours, or overnight, until the strawberries shrink and the flavors concentrate a bit. They should still be soft, but not as wet and watery as fresh berries.

3 Transfer the strawberries to a food processor, making sure to include all of the gooey concentrated strawberry juice from the Teflex sheet—you may need to use a spatula to get all of this concentrated jelly flavor. Add the stevia, if using, and pulse a few times to make a jam. Transfer to a covered container and store in the refrigerator until ready to use.

4 Place the almond butter, honey, and salt in a small bowl and mix well to combine.

5 Spread the honey nut butter on half of the bread slices. Top with strawberry jam, and the remaining bread slices.

Cinnamon-Date French Toast

with bananas, walnuts, and maple syrup

SERVES 4

You may want to drink the milk after soaking the bread in it. It's very sweet and tasty and it would be a shame to throw it out. You can use any kind of Manna bread, but some are less sweet than the cinnamon date, so you may want to adjust accordingly.

> "This isn't exactly like the crispy and fluffy French toast you might make with egg-soaked brioche and lots of butter in a pan, but honestly, eating that kind is not even remotely appealing anymore and would just make me feel gross. To me, this is a really tasty indulgence that is (of course) good for you! It's a nice thing to make for a cold weather brunch." —MK

For the French toast:

1 loaf Cinnamon Date Manna bread, cut into 12 slices about ¹/₂ inch thick (see Sources, page 360)

3 cups almond milk or Brazil nut milk (pages 52 and 57)

¹/₂ cup maple syrup

1 tablespoon ground cinnamon

¹/₂ teaspoon freshly ground nutmeg

¹/₂ teaspoon sea salt

1 Place the bread slices in a shallow baking dish. In a medium mixing bowl, whisk together the nut milk, maple syrup, cinnamon, nutmeg, and salt. Pour over the bread slices to cover. Move the pieces of bread around to make sure they are being soaked on all sides. Allow to soak for about an hour. You may want to flip them over halfway through

2 Let the milk drain off each slice, discard or drink the milk, and transfer the soaked bread to Teflex-lined dehydrator trays and dehydrate at 115°F for 4 to 6 hours, or until the tops are dry. Flip them over onto dehydrator screens and dehydrate further for approximately 4 more hours, or until dry and slightly crisp on both sides.

3 If you make these ahead of time and refrigerate (for up to a day or two), return them to the dehydrator for at least an hour before serving, to warm them through and recrisp.

For serving:

2 ripe bananas, sliced

¹/₂ cup Candied Walnuts (see page 294)

³/₄ cup maple syrup

Place 3 slices on each of 4 plates. Top with sliced bananas, candied walnuts, and maple syrup. Serve warm.

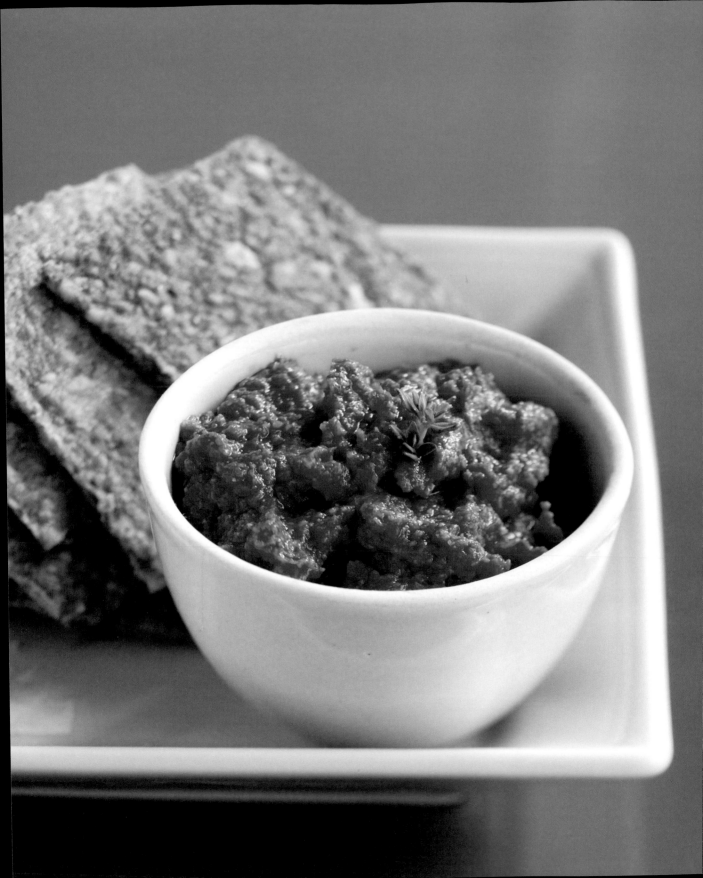

CHEESES, SPICED NUTS, CRACKERS, AND CONDIMENTS

This is the chapter you want to refer to when you're hungry. Or, more to the point, when you want to prevent being hungry. Let's face it, we all love to snack.

Plus, a large part of the raw food lifestyle is about being prepared, so that when you are in the mood to graze you choose something that is good for you.

If you think you might miss dairy products, especially cheese, pay attention. Many raw food books recommend Rejuvelac™, which is a fermented wheat berry liquid that yields a cheese-like consistency (see page 287 for more information). Adding lemon juice and nutritional yeast to nut mixes provides a nice cheese flavor with far less work. Try varying these recipes with different fresh herbs or spices.

For the spiced and candied nuts, try your own variations—they are endless. Nuts are an excellent way to add crunch to salads or any other dish, and a nice garnish for desserts or creamy ice cream, and they are also an ideal snack. For some of the spiced or candied nut recipes that call for maple sugar, you can always use maple syrup, honey, agave nectar, or yacon syrup—but the drying process will just take a bit longer. These spiced or candied nuts or seeds keep well in a covered container, but will keep longer and stay crunchier if stored in the refrigerator.

For the crackers, use the recipes as a base. You can try making them using other nuts, and experiment with different herbs and spices for variation. These are easy to make and keep well.

Don't rely solely on this chapter for condiments, as we have only included a few here. You can pull some parts from other recipes and use as condiments. For example, all of the components from the Zucchini and Green Zebra Tomato Lasagne (page 173) are great used in other ways; either together or separately on crackers or as a spread on the pizza crust with avocado or other vegetables. The hummus from the Flatbread Pizza on page 216 is great on its own or with sliced vegetables, or just wrapped in romaine lettuce leaves. Feel free to get creative and experiment.

Sun-Dried Tomato and Cashew Romesco

MAKES ABOUT 8 CUPS

Romesco is a traditional Spanish sauce or spread usually made with nuts, roasted red peppers, and olive oil. Here we use sun-dried tomatoes and add our own seasonings. Sun-dried tomatoes were a trend in the nineties, but we still love them for their all-natural sweetness and the versatility they lend to recipes. You can make your own dried tomatoes in a dehydrator. When we first opened the restaurant, Louisa, one of our sous-chefs, made this to serve with sliced baby greenmarket vegetables.

2 cups sun-dried tomatoes, soaked 1 hour or more
2 cups raw cashews, soaked for 2 hours or more
Zest of 1 orange
³/₄ cup olive oil
³/₄ cup orange juice
¹/₂ cup lemon juice
¹/₄ cup red miso
1 small clove garlic, chopped
1 tablespoon za'atar seasoning
2 teaspoons sea salt
Freshly ground black pepper

Place all of the ingredients in a food processor and blend well until thoroughly combined. Add water if necessary to thin a bit for a soft, spreadable consistency, and adjust seasoning. Serve with crackers or sliced vegetables.

Pine Nut Parmesan

MAKES ABOUT 3 CUPS

Pine nuts, also called pinyon and pignoli, are harvested from pine cones. They are one of the mildest nuts that nature has to offer and are suitable for everything from garnishes to desserts. We like this cream-colored, thin, crispy cheese that tastes quite a bit like Parmesan.

This is really good crumbled on salads or any sort of raw 'pasta' dish, or left in shards and used to top vegetable carpaccios. It's also easy to want to just eat the whole recipe plain, so you might think about making a double batch to account for the 'tasting shortage,' which is what you lose by stopping by the dehydrator a little too often to taste it while it's drying.

2 cups raw pine nuts, soaked 1 hour or more
$^{1}/_{2}$ cup filtered water
$^{1}/_{4}$ cup lemon juice
2 tablespoons nutritional yeast
$^{1}/_{2}$ teaspoon sea salt

1 In a food processor, blend all the ingredients until smooth and creamy. Divide the mixture between two 14-inch Teflex-lined dehydrator trays. Using an offset spatula, spread very thin and dehydrate at 115°F for 6 to 8 hours, or overnight. Break into chards and flip over to dry undersides, another 1 to 2 hours.

2 Store in an airtight container. This will keep a few days at room temperature or up to 7 to 10 days if refrigerated. It can also be frozen.

Macadamia Cheese

MAKES ABOUT 3 CUPS

At 80 percent oil, macadamia nuts have garnered a reputation for being one of the most fattening nuts available. But that's precisely what makes the kernels so useful in this recipe; after all, dairy cheese is mostly fat. The monosaturated oil of macadamia nuts has also been getting quite a bit of press as being not only good for the heart, but a very effective metabolism booster as well. So make a double batch and eat this cheese without guilt! The nutritional yeast is not necessary, but it adds a bit of an extra cheesy flavor and some vitamin B_{12}, too.

This is really easy to make and it tastes surprisingly . . . cheesy. In fact, when you use red peppers, the color of the cheese comes eerily close to that unnaturally bright orange hue of Doritos. Whenever we make this at home, it doesn't last long because it's hard to stop eating it. It's really good on salads or on a pasta dish with a creamy sauce.

1 1/2 cups chopped red bell pepper

3 tablespoons lime juice

1 1/2 teaspoons sea salt

1 1/2 cups macadamia nuts

1 tablespoon nutritional yeast (optional)

In a blender, puree the red pepper, lime juice, and sea salt. Place the macadamia nuts in a food processor and pulse a few times to chop them. Pour the red pepper mixture over the nuts and process until well combined but still a tiny bit chunky. Spread to about 1/4-inch thickness on Teflex-lined dehydrator trays and dehydrate at 115°F for 4 to 6 hours, or overnight. Once the top has dried, break it into shards and flip over to dry the undersides, another 1 to 2 hours. Store in an airtight container for a few days or longer in the refrigerator or freezer. See if it lasts even a week before you eat it all.

YELLOW PEPPER MACADAMIA CHEESE Use yellow bell pepper in place of the red bell pepper and lemon juice in place of the lime juice. Adding 1/2 teaspoon of cumin gives it nice extra flavor as well.

Rejuvelac

Rejuvelac is a highly nutritious fermented liquid made simply from sprouted wheat berries which replenishes healthy intestinal flora—key for efficient digestion—and helps to restore your colon's pH balance, always a good thing. It was popularized by Ann Wigmore, considered by many to be among the most significant pioneers, teachers, and authors about healing with raw foods. You can actually use any grain to make Rejuvelac, but wheat berries seem to be most commonly recommended.

To make Rejuvelac, soak about 2 cups of soft wheat berries in water for 8 hours or overnight. Drain off and discard the water and let the wheat berries sprout for about 2 days, until the small white tails begin to grow. (To sprout, simply let the soaked grain sit in a fine-mesh colander at room temperature, covered with a clean towel.) Add the sprouted wheat berries to a large glass container with about a gallon of water, cover with cheesecloth or some other breathable cloth and secure it with a rubber band or string. Place it in a warm location—around 70°F is ideal—and let it sit for about 48 hours. It should become sour tasting and fizzy (it sounds gross, but it shouldn't taste gross—if it tastes *off*, get rid of it and start again). Drain the liquid into a separate container and add a tablespoon or two of lemon juice, which makes it taste better and helps to keep it fresh. You can reuse the wheat berries to make another batch, but use slightly less water and let the sprouted wheat sit for only 24 (not 48) hours. The best thing to do with the spent grains is to toss them out the kitchen window for birds as we do in Maine, but not, of course, in the city.

Rejuvelac keeps for about a week or so in the refrigerator. Some people, like live food gurus David Jubb and Annie Padden Jubb, recommend adding the powder from a capsule or two of acidopholous to the water with the wheat berries, which they says encourages the growth of more good bacterias, and also prevents "stinky-sock tasting Rejuvelac." Lovely, right? If you can get over the weirdness of fizzy liquids and any negative associations with fermentation, Rejuvelac is a great thing to add to your diet. You can use it to make cheeses, pureeing it with soaked nuts and letting it sit in a warm place, then straining out the liquid with cheesecloth. But it's easier and you get more out of it by just drinking it straight. When we first went raw, we always had some on hand and added some to fruit-based shakes, or mixed it with lots of lemon and lime juice and drank it over ice. It's especially good to have if you've been taking antibiotics or doing a lot of colonics, or just feel like doing something nice for your colon. Because who doesn't want a happy colon?

Fluffy Macadamia Feta

MAKES ABOUT 4 CUPS

This cheese accents the Warm Cherry Tomato and Sweet Corn Salad on page 119. You can always add fresh herbs directly to this cheese as well.

4 cups raw macadamia nuts, soaked 1 hour or more
1/4 cup lemon juice
2 tablespoons nutritional yeast

1 green onion, white and 1 inch green, minced
2 teaspoons sea salt

In a food processor, thoroughly grind all the ingredients, but leave it a bit chunky. Drop heaping teaspoonfuls onto Teflex-lined dehydrator trays and dehydrate at 115°F for 4 to 6 hours, or until dry on the outside and still tender on the inside. Store in an airtight container in the refrigerator for up to a week or so.

Candied Pumpkin Seeds

MAKES 2 CUPS

Flat, dark green pumpkin seeds (pepitas) are a great high-protein snack. Rich in zinc, they are also particularly vital for men's health, containing elements that help protect the prostrate and bones. Pumpkin seeds go nicely on a fall salad or to garnish desserts.

2 cups pumpkin seeds, soaked 4 hours or more
1 tablespoon ground ginger

1/4 cup maple syrup powder (see Sources, page 360)
1/2 teaspoon fine sea salt

Drain the pumpkin seeds very well and place in a medium bowl with the remaining ingredients. Toss well to combine. Spread on a dehydrator tray. Dehydrate at 115°F for 12 to 24 hours, or until dry and crisp.

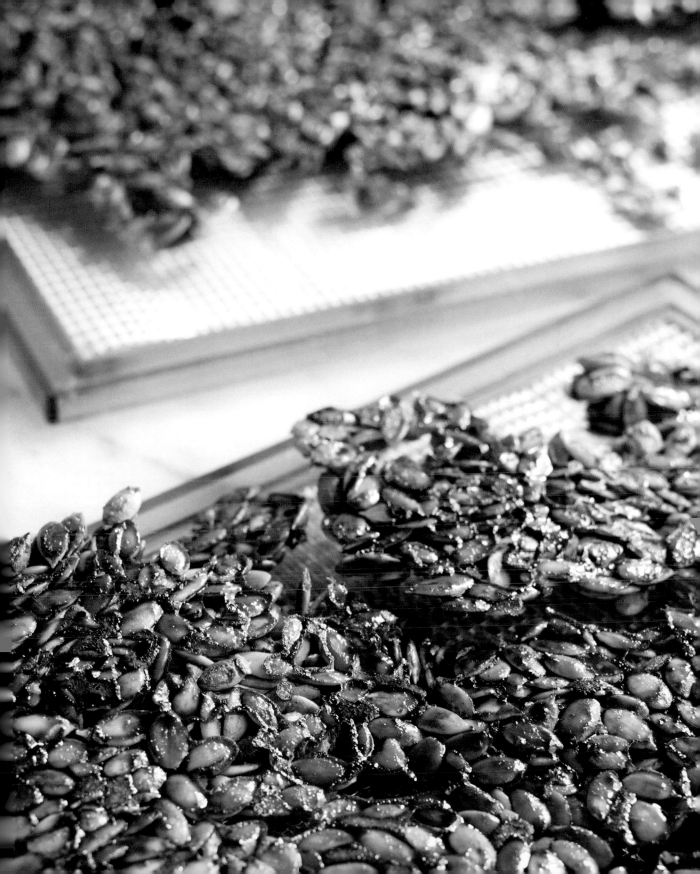

Spicy Chili Lime Almonds

MAKES 4 CUPS

We like these because they have so much flavor—whenever they are being made in the restaurant it's hard to keep our hands out of the dehydrator. They are a really good snack on their own.

4 cups almonds, soaked for 6 hours or more
¹/₂ cup agave nectar
¹/₄ cup maple sugar or date sugar (see Sources, page 363)
¹/₄ cup lime juice
2 tablespoons chile powder
2 tablespoons ground fennel
1 tablespoon sea salt

Drain the almonds well and place them in a large bowl with the remaining ingredients. Toss well to coat. Pour the nuts onto two 14-inch Teflex-lined dehydrator sheets, making sure to pour any remaining juices and seasoning onto the nuts. Dehydrate at 115°F for 3 to 4 hours, or until most liquid on tray is dried. Transfer the nuts onto unlined screens and dehydrate overnight, or until crisp.

Spiced Brazil Nuts

MAKES 2 CUPS

Brazil nut trees are the only commercial ones that have stubbornly refused to be cultivated on plantations or in groves. As such, they live exclusively in the Amazonian rainforest, where they can produce for more than 1,000 years. But falling prices in the world nut market and a lack of popularity tempt the Peruvians and Brazilians who harvest them to slash-and-burn the forests and plant better income-producing crops. So don't bother hugging a tree, just eat more Brazil nuts, and you could play a role in saving the rainforest.

I love snacking on these or tossing them in a salad, especially because Brazil nuts are so rich-tasting and nutritious, and other than in our nut milks, we don't eat enough of them.

2 cups Brazil nuts, soaked for 1 hour or more, thinly sliced
²/₃ cup agave nectar or raw honey
2 teaspoons ground chile powder
1 generous pinch sea salt

In a medium bowl, mix the sliced Brazil nuts with the agave nectar, chile powder, and a generous pinch of salt, tossing to coat the nuts. Spread the nuts on a Teflex-lined dehydrator tray and dehydrate at 115°F for 24 to 48 hours. The longer they dehydrate, the crunchier they will be.

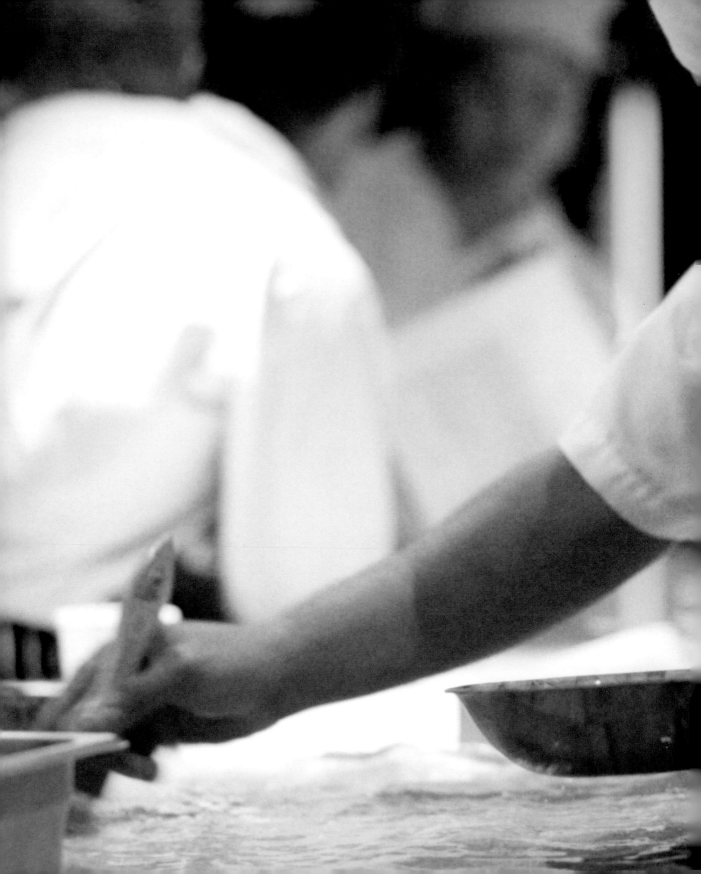

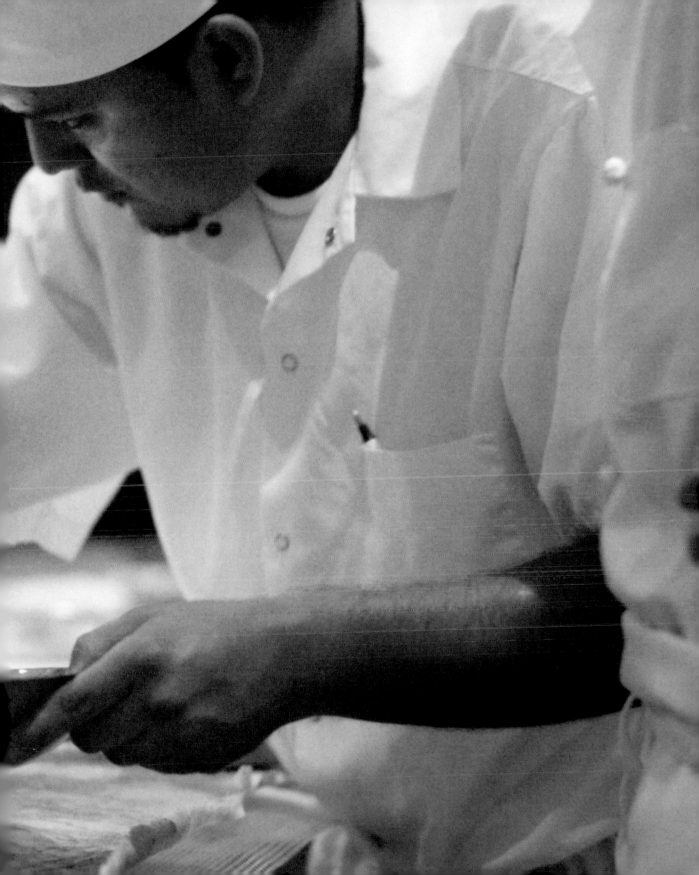

Maple-Sugared Slivered Almonds

MAKES 4 CUPS

These are *really* nice folded into our Vanilla Ice Cream (page 253), or sprinkled on the Chocolate Pudding (page 239).

4 cups slivered raw almonds, soaked for
    30 minutes or more
1 cup maple syrup powder (see Sources, page 364)

1/2 teaspoon ground chili powder
2 teaspoons sea salt

Drain the almonds well and place them in a large bowl with the remaining ingredients and toss well to coat. Pour the nuts onto two 14-inch Teflex-lined dehydrator sheets and dehydrate at 115°F for 6 to 8 hours, or until crisp.

Candied Walnuts

MAKES 4 CUPS

Try these in a banana split. Slice some bananas, top with Vanilla Ice Cream (page 253) and some freshly made ganache and vanilla cream from the Dark Chocolate Ganache Tart (page 231), and these walnuts.

4 cups coarsely chopped walnuts, soaked
    for 1 hour or more
1/2 cup maple syrup powder (see Sources, page 364)

1/2 cup agave nectar
1 teaspoon ground cinnamon
2 teaspoons fine sea salt

In a medium bowl, toss the walnuts with the maple sugar, agave nectar, cinnamon, and salt. Spread the nuts on two 14-inch Teflex-lined dehydrator trays and dehydrate at 115°F for 12 hours or more, until crisp.

Walnut Hemp Crackers

MAKES ABOUT 48 3-INCH CRACKERS

Made with walnuts, flax, and hemp, this flatbread is rich in vitamin E and omega-3 (walnuts have more omega-3 fatty acids than any nut) and also a good source of protein. These are chewy and yummy, though you could spread the mix a bit more thinly over four trays instead of three for crisper crackers. We cut them in long, thin triangles and serve them with the Tomato Tartare (page 146) at the restaurant.

5 cups walnuts, soaked 1 hour or more
5 cups diced zucchini
³/₄ cup golden flaxseed, finely ground
  (about 1 cup ground)

¹/₂ cup hemp seeds
¹/₄ to ¹/₂ cup filtered water
1 tablespoon sea salt

1   In a food processor, add the walnuts and grind to a fine texture, but try not to overprocess to a paste. Transfer the nuts to a large bowl. Add the zucchini to the same food processor bowl and grind well. Add the zucchini to the walnuts as well as the flaxseeds and hemp seeds, stirring to combine. Add water, as necessary, until a sticky dough forms—like wet muffin batter. Season with the sea salt, adding more or less to taste.

2   Divide the batter between three 14-inch Teflex-lined dehydrator trays. Using an offset spatula, spread the dough to the edges of the trays. The dough can be a bit gummy and sticky, so it helps to dip the spatula in water as you spread it (the excess water will evaporate in the dehydrator).

3   Dehydrate the flatbread at 115°F for 6 to 8 hours, or overnight. When the tops are dry, flip them over and peel away the liners. Dehydrate further for another 2 to 3 hours or longer.

4   Once both sides are dry, slide the flatbread onto a large cutting board. Cut into squares, rectangles, or any shape. Place them back on the dehydrator trays and dehydrate another hour or two, until crisp. Store in an airtight container for about a week, or longer in the refrigerator.

Sun-Dried Tomato and Herb Crackers

MAKES 64 3-INCH CRACKERS

This is really just a variation on the Walnut Hemp Crackers. The addition of sun-dried tomatoes, herbs, and other ingredients gives the recipe a zestier flavor that helps the crackers stand on their own.

5 cups walnuts, soaked 1 hour or more
5 cups diced zucchini
1 large handful sun-dried tomatoes, soaked at least 1 hour
1 small handful oregano, marjoram, or other herbs
4 to 5 green onions, roughly chopped
³/₄ cup golden flaxseed, finely ground (about 1 cup ground)
¹/₂ cup hemp seeds
¹/₃ cup lemon juice
¹/₃ cup nutritional yeast
¹/₄ to ¹/₂ cup filtered water
1 tablespoon sea salt

1 In a food processor, add the walnuts and grind to a fine texture, but try not to overprocess to a paste. Transfer the nuts to a large bowl. Add the zucchini to the same food processor bowl with the tomatoes, herbs, and green onions and grind well. Add the zucchini mixture to the walnuts. Add the flaxseeds, hemp seeds, lemon juice, and yeast, stirring to combine. Add water, as necessary, until a sticky dough forms—like wet muffin batter. Season with the sea salt, adding more or less to taste.

2 Divide the batter between four 14-inch Teflex-lined dehydrator trays and proceed as for the Walnut Hemp Crackers (page 295).

Jalapeño Corn Tortilla Chips

MAKES 48 3-INCH CRACKERS

Pair these with salsa and guacamole from the Soft Corn Tortilla recipe (page 188). This is one of our favorite snacks.

3 cups fresh corn from 2–3 ears
$1^{1}/_{2}$ cups chopped yellow or red bell pepper
$^{1}/_{2}$ small yellow onion
$^{3}/_{4}$ cup golden flaxseed, finely ground (about 1 cup ground)
$^{1}/_{2}$ cup hemp seeds
2 tablespoons lime juice
1 to 2 jalapeño peppers, minced, seeds to taste
$^{1}/_{2}$ teaspoon ground chili powder
2 teaspoons ground cumin
2 teaspoons sea salt

1 In a food processor, chop the corn, bell pepper, and onion until smooth. Add the remaining ingredients and process until just combined.

2 Using an offset spatula, spread the dough thinly onto three 14-inch Teflex-lined dehydrator trays. Dehydrate at 115°F for 6 to 8 hours, or overnight. Flip the sheets over onto the tray and carefully peel away the liners. Break or cut into pieces. Place back in the dehydrator for 4 to 6 hours, or until crisp. Store in an airtight container for a week or two.

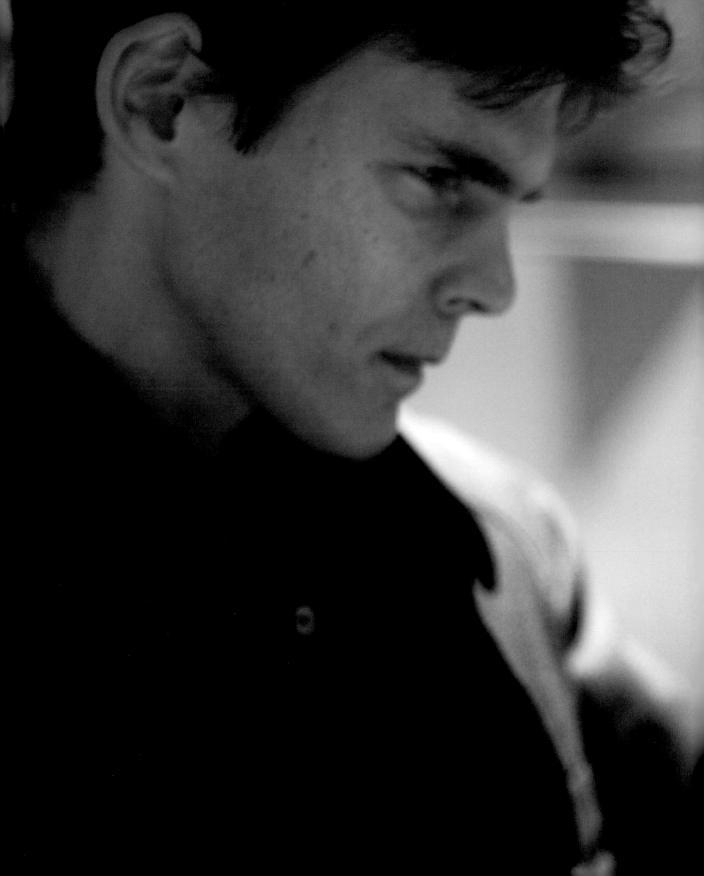

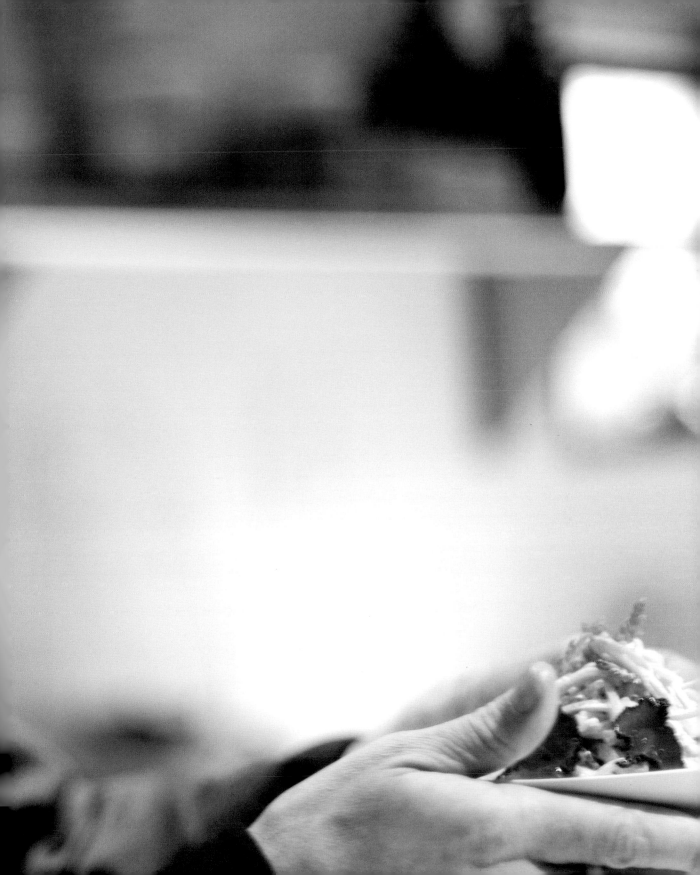

Spicy Flax and Herb Crackers

MAKES ABOUT 64 3-INCH CRACKERS

Flaxseeds are mini powerhouses of essential fatty acids. You can also try soaking the seeds whole overnight and then incorporating them into the recipe that way—they will get a bit gelatinous and make a crisp cracker. But we like the texture of ground flax best and think its goodness is more easily assimilated this way. If you like you can substitute regular flaxseeds for the golden flax.

1 cup sunflower seeds, soaked 1 hour or more

1 cup raw almonds, soaked 2 hours or more

$1/2$ cup sun-dried tomatoes, soaked 1 hour or more

2 red bell peppers, cored and chopped

3 to 4 small jalapeño peppers, cored

2 cups golden flaxseeds, finely ground (about $2^2/3$ cup ground)

$1/2$ cup lime juice

1 tablespoon cumin powder

1 tablespoon chili powder

1 tablespoon sea salt

1 large handful mixed fresh herbs, such as cilantro, basil, and parsley

1 In a food processor, place the sunflower seeds, almonds, and tomatoes and pulse to chop. Add the red bell and jalapeño peppers, flaxseed, lime juice, cumin, chili powder, and salt and process to combine well. Add water if needed to thin to a spreadable consistency. Taste for seasoning, add fresh herbs, and pulse to chop and incorporate.

2 Using an offset spatula, spread the dough thinly onto four 14-inch Teflex-lined dehydrator trays. Dehydrate at 115°F for 6 to 8 hours, or overnight. Flip the sheets over onto the tray and carefully peel away the liners. Break or cut into pieces. Place back in the dehydrator for 4 to 6 hours, or until crispy. Store in an airtight container for up to a week or two.

Mango Chutney

MAKES ABOUT 4 CUPS

We pair this with the Cauliflower Samosas (page 204), but it's a nice accompaniment to other dishes and great on its own as well.

I love mangos. Adding the tart lime, ginger, and savory flavors of green onion and jalapeño cuts the sweetness. Unlike many other fruits, mangos work really well with heat and spice and often appear in many exotic dishes.

4 cups diced ripe mango
3 tablespoons lime juice
2 tablespoons minced ginger
2 green onions, white and 1 inch of green, diced
1/2 small jalapeño, cored and seeded, diced
1/2 teaspoon sea salt
1 small handful cilantro leaves

In a food processor, add all of the ingredients and pulse to combine well, but keep it chunky. Store in a covered container in the refrigerator for up to 2 to 3 days.

Green Olive Tapenade

MAKES 3 ½ CUPS

We make this tapenade for the Flatbread Pizza, but it's also great served plain with crackers.

Years ago when I opened my first restaurant, Matthew's, a different version of green olive tapenade was one of the first recipes we wrote (to go with tuna tartare and fennel). At the time it was unusual to use milder green olives rather than the more common black olives in tapenade.

3 cups pitted green olives
½ cup extra virgin olive oil
2 tablespoons lemon juice
1 small handful parsley (optional)
Freshly ground black pepper

1 Process the olives in a food processor. With the motor running, add the olive oil and lemon juice and process until smooth. Add the parsley (if using) and process to combine. Season with pepper to taste.

2 Transfer to a covered container and refrigerate. Will keep up to 1 to 2 weeks.

Tart Sour Cream

MAKES ABOUT 3 CUPS

Top Jalapeño Corn Tortilla Chips (page 297) with guacamole, salsa, diced olives, Macadamia Cheese (page 286), and a drizzle of this cream for a big plate of soul-satisfying "nachos."

I've always loved sour cream with fruits
and other desserts. Tart and sweet is always
a nice combination.

1 cup coconut meat
3 tablespoons lemon juice
2 tablespoons apple cider vinegar
1 tablespoon white miso paste
1 cup filtered water
$^1/_2$ cup cashew nuts, soaked for about 1 to 2 hours
1 teaspoon sea salt

In a blender, blend the coconut meat with the lemon juice, cider vinegar, miso, and $^1/_2$ cup of the water until smooth. Add the soaked cashews and more water, 1 tablespoon at a time and blend until completely smooth (you may need more than 1 cup of water). Season with salt and blend further. Transfer to a squeeze bottle or covered container and refrigerate until ready to use. Can be kept for up to 2 or 3 days.

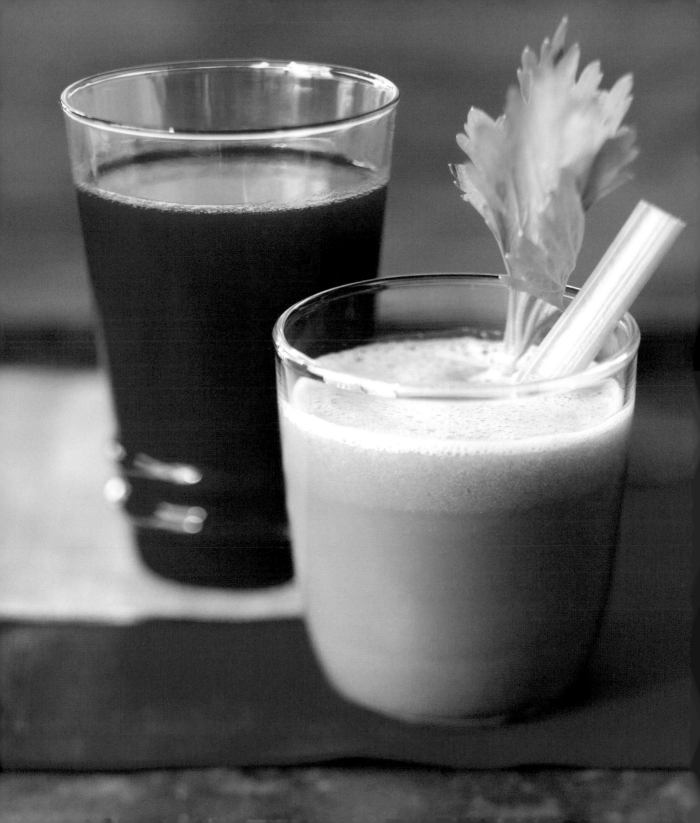

JUICES

Think of juices as liquid vitamin supplements, only better tasting. They
are concentrated nutrition, the
FedEx of foods—a delivery service
that gets there in half the time.
Juices give the body a break from
the arduous process of digestion,

which is why they are great for cleansing; the nutrients, packed with antioxidants and essential amino acids, are rapidly assimilated. If there's one thing that has the most positive and immediate impact on your health, it's drinking organic green juices daily.

Okay, that's the glass-half-full look at juicing. The reality is that it can be quite messy and time-consuming to do at home. If you have the space, get a good juicer, even if you don't use it every day. We bought our juicer and had tons of fun experimenting with it and making lots of juices in the beginning, but we also were lucky enough to have some leisure time. Eventually, we found a great organic juice bar not far from where we live and our own juicer got tucked away in a cupboard. Luckily, juice bars are sprouting up all over. Just be sure to find one that uses only organic produce. Now, of course, we are spoiled by our restaurant's own juice bar!

Juicing is very much like making shakes. You don't really need to measure, and there are endless combinations you can make. The fun part is looking in the fridge or on the counter and seeing what you can run through the juicer! Don't overlook what you might think of as waste for the compost pile, either. For example, watermelon rinds are great for you—all the good stuff is concentrated near the skin.

Just remember to always use organic produce, especially when you'll be juicing the peel, skin, or seeds. Cut the fruits, such as apples and pears, into manageable pieces that will fit through your juicer. When you use lemons, cut away the outer yellow peel, but leave on some of the white pith—it's great for you. Drink fresh juice as soon as possible after you've made it (or purchased it from a juice bar)—the nutrients lose their value pretty quickly once they are exposed to oxygen.

Basic Green

SERVES 2

When juicing greens and herbs, the fibers sometimes get caught and it becomes difficult to push them through. We've found that it helps to alternate greens with the celery
and apple. Or chop up the greens, celery, and apple, toss all together in a bowl and add it
to the juicer in batches.

> "Sarma and I have a 16-ounce green juice almost every day,
> sometimes more than one a day. Drinking pure green juice can
> be an acquired taste. We didn't really love it at first. But add
> lots of lemon or lime, and start out mixing it with apple or a bit
> of fresh ginger, or both. Now I crave it more than anything,
> and love the way it makes me feel. It really is like giving your
> body the purest fuel." —MK

8 to 10 large leaves kale, collards, swiss chard, or a combination
¹/₂ **bunch parsley**
3 stalks celery
¹/₂ **apple**
¹/₂ **lemon, outer yellow peel cut away**

Run all ingredients through a juicer.

Fruit Spice

SERVES 2

This is a basic, refreshing juice that is great served over ice. You can also cut the pineapple core into thin strips to use as stirrers.

¼ **medium pineapple**
2 ripe pears, such as Anjou
1 thumb-size knob fresh ginger

Run all ingredients through a juicer. Pour over ice and serve.

Thai Green

SERVES 2

Cilantro is known to help pull toxic metals out of our bodies. It's also an essential herb found in many world cuisines, from Vietnamese to Mexican, which have become more popular in the past decade.

"I love cilantro—I could eat a whole salad of it, so this is one of my favorite ways to drink greens. —SM"

6 to 8 large leaves kale, collards, swiss chard, or a combination
1 small bunch cilantro
¼ **medium pineapple**
2 limes, outer peel cut away and discarded

Run all ingredients through a juicer.

Hot Pink

Beets are rich in folate and folic acid, especially good for pregnant women. Known as nature's multivitamin. If you find beets with the tops still attached, reserve them for a salad—beet greens are even more nutritious than their roots.

1 medium beet, peeled
¹/₂ medium pineapple
¹/₂ pint strawberries, stems removed
1 thumb-size knob fresh ginger

Run all ingredients through a juicer.

Spicy Skin Saver

This drink is like having a facial from the inside out. Radishes and watercress are especially rich in sulfur, which helps to build collagen, a nutrient that's necessary for elasticity. Grape seeds are full of essential fatty oils and antioxidants that protect the skin against free radical damage. And cucumbers keep you well hydrated, a must for good skin!

¹/₂ cup chopped radish
6 cups green grapes, preferably seeded
¹/₂ bunch watercress, or 4 to 5 large kale leaves
1 large cucumber
1 very small knob fresh ginger

Run all ingredients through a juicer.

Cucumber Mint Cooler

SERVES 2

Cucumbers are hydrating and cooling, and a good diuretic. They help to flush wastes through the kidneys and dissolve uric acid accumulations such as kidney and bladder stones. Celery also contains a lot of natural sodium to help keep you hydrated.

" **This is really good in the summertime over a lot of ice.** " —MK

2 medium cucumbers
2 stalks celery
1 small handful fresh mint, plus additional for garnish
2 limes, outer peel cut away and discarded

1 Run all ingredients through a juicer.

2 Pour over ice and garnish with mint sprigs.

Free Rads and Anti-Oxes

Free radicals may sound like terrorists that have eluded capture and are bent on wreaking havoc, and in fact that's a pretty apt comparison. Free radicals are molecules gone awry. They evolve when a molecule's bonds are split inappropriately and its electrons distributed unevenly. The free radical, lacking a balancing electron, then latches onto any other compound in search of an electron to steal, and it doesn't discriminate. The molecule it cons then becomes a free radical itself. And they tell two friends, and they tell two friends, and so on . . .

Some free radicals occur naturally through metabolism, and others are caused by external factors including pollution, cigarette smoke, and radiation. Cooking food forms many free radicals because heating breaks down molecular structure. When enough free radicals form in a single living cell, the immune system is beckoned. But like any reproducing virus or bacteria, the more free radicals present, the harder they are to fight. Furthermore, if the immune system is weakened from the outset or engaged in battle elsewhere, damage will occur.

Enter antioxidants. Antioxidants, absorbed naturally by the body in the form of fruit and plant vitamins, sacrifice one of their own electrons to free radicals, which stop them from feasting on other molecules. Antioxidants don't become free radicals themselves because their molecular make-up is stable in any form. Call them the ground troops, expendable heroes who fight dirty to keep our bodies clean. But they still need to be drafted, so eat your fruits and veggies raw, as nature intended.

Time to Go

SERVES 2

Yes, you can take that as a bad pun. But this juice is indeed good for when the train has been a bit late pulling out of the station. This is not a common affliction on a diet of raw foods, which generally keeps our internal Amtrak moving along quite regularly, but occasionally we all need a little help! Some fruits like pears, apples, and prunes have high levels of sorbitol, a naturally occurring, nondigestible form of sugar that pulls water into the intestines. As an added bonus, prunes are also particularly high in iron.

> **This juice is not a particularly lovely color, but it tastes surprisingly good—so be careful not to drink *too* much.** —SM

8 to 10 large leaves kale, collards, swiss chard, or a combination
4 pears or apples
4 to 6 pitted prunes

Run all ingredients through a juicer.

Honeymoon Healer

SERVES 2

As many females know, drinking cranberry juice is the ultimate protection against urinary tract infections (also commonly known as the honeymoon disease, given the reasons why it usually flares up). Most Western doctors treat it by prescribing antibiotics, which unfortunately kill all the healthy bacteria and only make one even more prone to future infections. Prevent the pain in the first place by drinking plenty of cranberry juice, especially at the beginning of a serious romantic relationship! Cranberries are also full of vitamin C and potassium.

2 cups fresh or frozen cranberries
1 lime, outer peel cut away and discarded
2 cups fresh orange juice
1 to 2 heaping tablespoons raw honey
1 lime, cut into very thin slices for garnish (optional)

1 Run the cranberries and lime through the juicer and stir into the orange juice.

2 Stir in the honey. If the honey is more solid than liquid, as raw honey usually is, pour a small amount of the juice into a glass or bowl and stir or whisk it together with the honey until it dissolves, then add it to the rest of the juice.

3 Pour over ice, add lime slices, if desired, and stir.

Blue-Green Algae

It certainly sounds a trifle unappetizing, like something you might scrape off the walls of your swimming pool. But blue-green algae, also known as Aphanizomenon flos-aquae (AFA), which sounds even worse to us, is an amazing substance. Harvested from Oregon's Klamath Lake, one of the only places in the United States where it grows naturally, wild blue-green algae is an incredible source of protein and chlorophyll (live enzymes!) as well as the hard to come by vitamin B_{12}. It is also said to induce immune cell production. Even more stimulating is the algae's emotional effect. According to the homepage of E3Live www.e3live.com, a wild food supermarket, the phenylethylamine (PEA) contained in AFA is referred to as the "molecule of love." While it may seem contra-indicative, blue-green algae also calms the nervous system, inspires focus, and increases attention span. Could this be a neat replacement for Ritalin? You can take blue-green algae in liquid form but as it needs to be stored frozen, it may not always be convenient. We also recommend the flake form or capsules; in addition to the liquid E3Live, we carry the Ancient Sun brand of flakes and capsules in our take-out store. See Sources, page 362, for information on where to get blue-green algae.

Blue Grape

SERVES 2 TO 4

This drink is a funky color from the blue-green algae. You don't need a vegetable juicer for this—just squeeze the grapefruits by hand (we use one of those knobby wooden tools that you hold, available in any cookware store). Grapefruit is an excellent cleanser of toxins.

> **This is my all-time favorite drink, especially first thing in the morning. At the restaurant, the grapefruit juice we use has been strained of pulp so you can drink it with a straw. At home, we keep all the pulp in it and usually end up eating it with a spoon.** —SM

2 tablespoons blue-green algae (flakes or liquid)
3 tablespoons agave or 2 packets stevia
4 cups freshly squeezed grapefruit juice

Stir the blue-green algae and sweetener into the grapefruit juice.

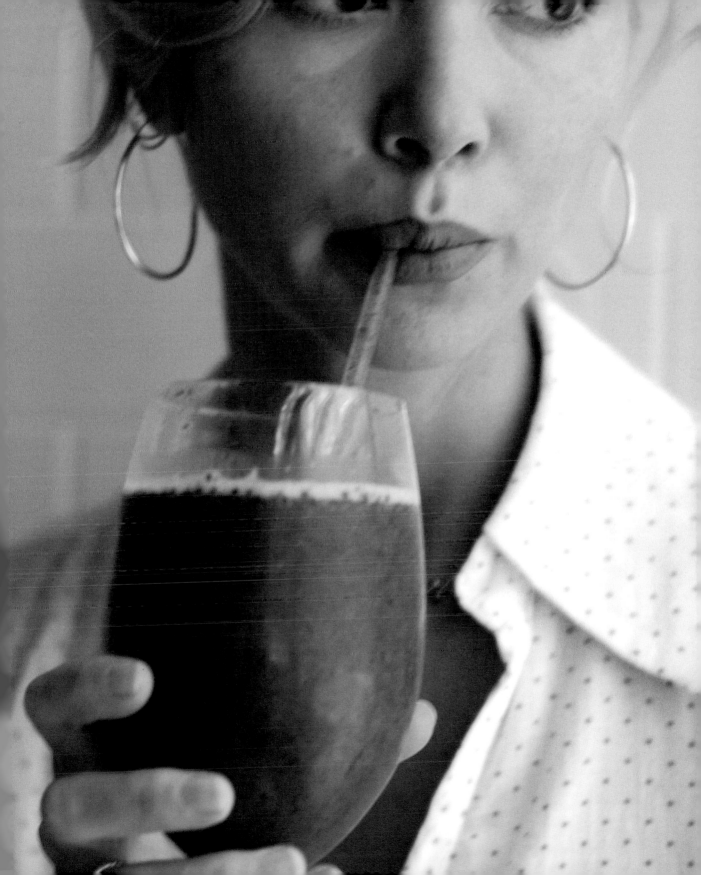

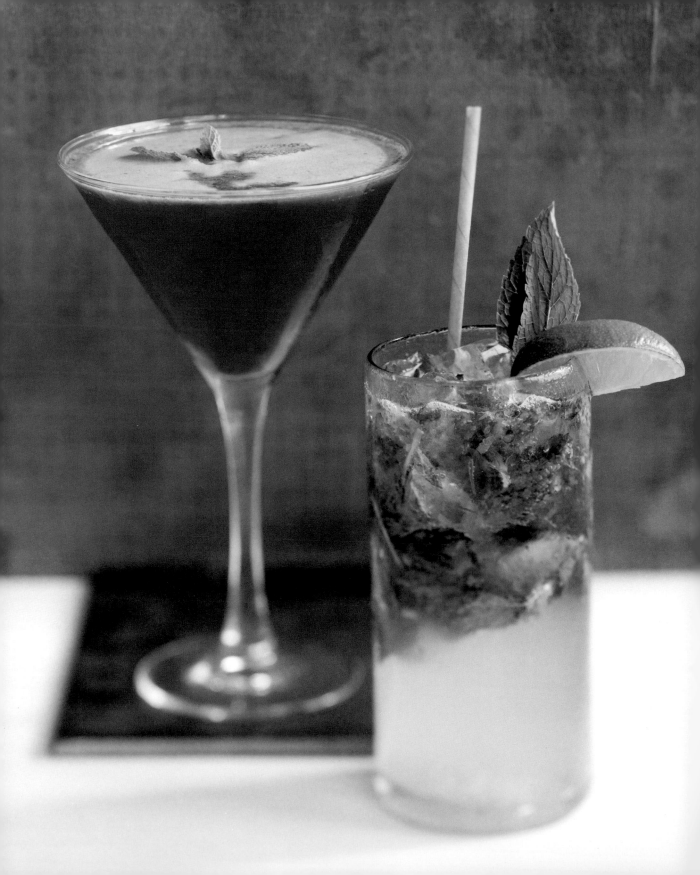

COCKTAILS

The clean, natural ingredients used in raw foods are perfectly suited to cocktails, especially during the summer. At Pure Food and Wine, our creative bartenders always keep us busy testing their latest version of these tasty drinks.

While sparkling and still wine are the bases for some of our specialty cocktails, organic sake is the main ingredient in many of our favorites. It should be noted that the sake we use, although organic and unpasteurized, is produced from rice that is first steamed. (See Sexy Sake page 325.)

These refreshing drinks are much better when served cold. It helps to have wine, champagne, or sake that has been thoroughly chilled before mixing it with the other ingredients.

As with most of our recipes, you can use these as guidelines and get creative with other ingredients, depending on the time of year. Feel free to adjust the amount of ingredients to suit whatever preferences you may have by adding more agave, citrus, or even sake. As always, use the best ingredients you can find, fully ripe and in their peak season. In the fall, we make a drink with fresh Concord grape juice (from the greenmarket) mixed with sake and champagne. In the summer when peaches are in season, we make Bellinis, which are amazing with white peaches.

These drinks, although good on their own, are designed to complement the subtleties of raw food and are all light and refreshing, not pungent or strong. Just don't be fooled by their pure, innocent flavors. A cautionary note: eating raw foods on an exclusive basis makes your tolerance for any sort of alcohol go way down. So where three or four glasses of wine, champagne, or cocktails might have made you feel nice and warm in the past, you may find yourself giddy after just two (or one!).

Pure Mojito

SERVES 2

Although we have nothing against a traditional mojito, the raw food pantry does not include rum, which is boiled and reduced to fermented sugar. We'll save you the hangover! This version is so clean and light tasting, and you won't get that residual, morning-after sugar effect.

> This is my favorite drink at the restaurant—I love lime and mint with anything. The hard part is not drinking too much, especially when it's warm out. —SM

1 big handful mint leaves
1 cup lime juice
¼ cup agave nectar
1 cup sake
1 cup ice cubes
1 cup champagne or sparkling white wine

Using the back of a spoon, mash the mint in the bottom of a pitcher or shaker with the lime juice and agave nectar. Divide between two rocks glasses. Add the sake and ice and stir. Top with champagne and serve with a straw.

Pink Spice Martini

SERVES 4

Don't let the beet juice scare you—it provides an extra hint of sweetness and the bright pink color. Like many of our cocktails, the flavors of the fruit often mask the taste of the sake, making it easy to drink a few too many.

Shortly after we opened the restaurant one night, after the kitchen had quieted down, I had a Pink Spice Martini. Then I sat at the bar in the garden with a friend and had another. It was so refreshing and sweet that I must not have noticed that the bartender kept giving me refills. Once Matthew and I stepped out to leave, I realized I'd had far too many. By the time we got home, I was feeling very insecure being anywhere other than by the cool tile of my bathroom floor, which is where I stubbornly insisted on sleeping, asking Matthew only to bring me a blanket and pillow. When I woke up early the next morning, I rolled over and there he was, asleep next to me on the floor. —SM

1 1/2 cups fresh green apple juice
1/2 cup fresh pear juice
3/4 cup sake
1/4 cup fresh beet juice
Splash of fresh ginger juice
4 cinnamon sticks

In a martini shaker, pour all the ingredients except the cinnamon sticks over ice and shake or stir very well to chill. Strain and pour into martini glasses and garnish with cinnamon sticks.

Red Sangria

SERVES 4

As the summer faded, Joey, one of our bartenders, developed this colorful alternative to our white sangria. The cayenne is a warming agent and, along with cinnamon, ginger, and the agave, it makes this a perfect autumn drink. We love the ruby red richness of this, especially when it is poured into a big round wine goblet.

1 bottle red wine, preferably Merlot, or another varietal with soft tannins
1 cinnamon stick
1 thumb-size knob ginger, cut into 2 or 3 slices, lengthwise
$1/4$ cup agave nectar
$1/4$ cup lemon juice
Pinch of cayenne pepper
1 red apple, cored and chopped
1 orange, sliced, seeds removed, and chopped
1 Anjou or Comice pear, diced
1 cup diced pineapple

1 In a large pitcher, mix all ingredients and refrigerate, covered, for a few hours or overnight.

2 To serve, remove the cinnamon stick and pieces of ginger and discard. Pour the sangria over ice in large wine goblets and servee with a spoon.

Sexy Sake

Like maple syrup, sake is not technically raw. It is fermented from steamed rice, yeast, a mold called *koji,* and water. Sake is also usually pasteurized.

We like it anyway, for several reasons: it's rich in amino acids; its beer-like, back-of-palate qualities allow it to pair beautifully with raw foods; and in recent years, many sake makers have ventured into organic growing and brewing processes. You can even get some sake that is unpasteurized (this is what we generally use, and it must be kept in the fridge).

There's a philosophy behind sake making, a treasured piece of Japanese culture, and a spiritual connection between the quaff and the quaffer. According to Benihana founder and sake expert Rocky Aoki, "Sake, with its four ingredients, is a very natural product. And to the Japanese, the human body is the ultimate natural product."

Sake has quite a reputation as a love potion. In his book *Saké: Water from Heaven, Aoki* theorizes that sake "is made to be sipped, not 'downed.' It is served in small cups that have to be refilled many times . . . the methodology of drinking sake is a major component of its enjoyment." He notes a similarity to sex. "The concept of the 'quickie' is certainly not Japanese. Sex in Japan is something to savor for its

Certainly the wine releases inhibitions: "Most Japanese homes are literally paper thin, offering lovers very little in terms of privacy. It is almost impossible to make love to your partner without everyone else in the family (and possibly some neighbors) knowing what you are doing. But after a few cups of sake, couples start to forget the reality of their surroundings and enjoy their union without embarrassment," Aoki writes. Yet another way to "get the glow."

Of course, drink too much and you'll be looking through sake goggles, so don't blame us if the world—or your partner in cocktail misdemeanors—looks a little bit less sexy the morning after. The good news, at any rate, is that sake generally doesn't give you a hangover.

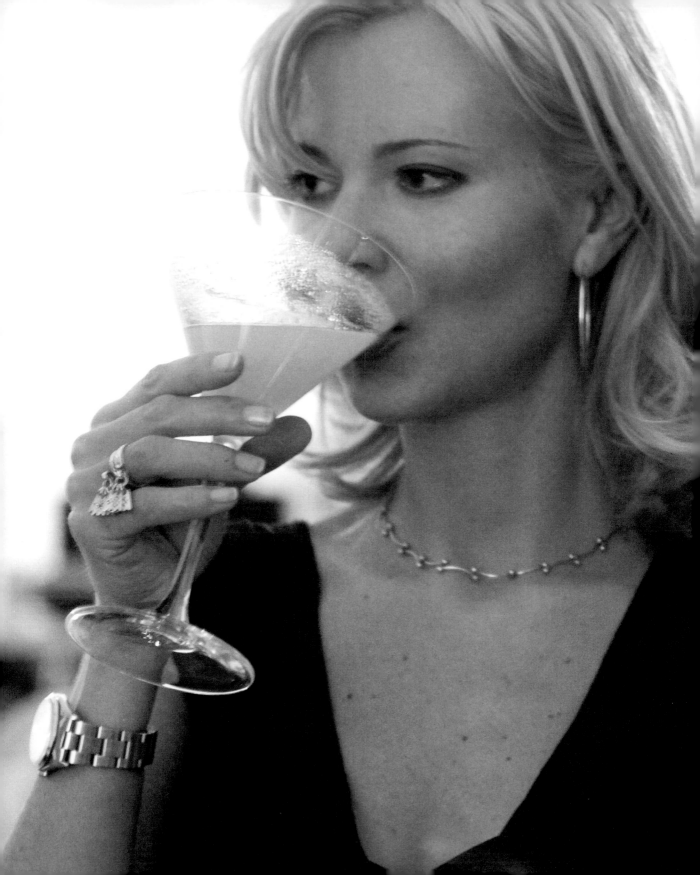

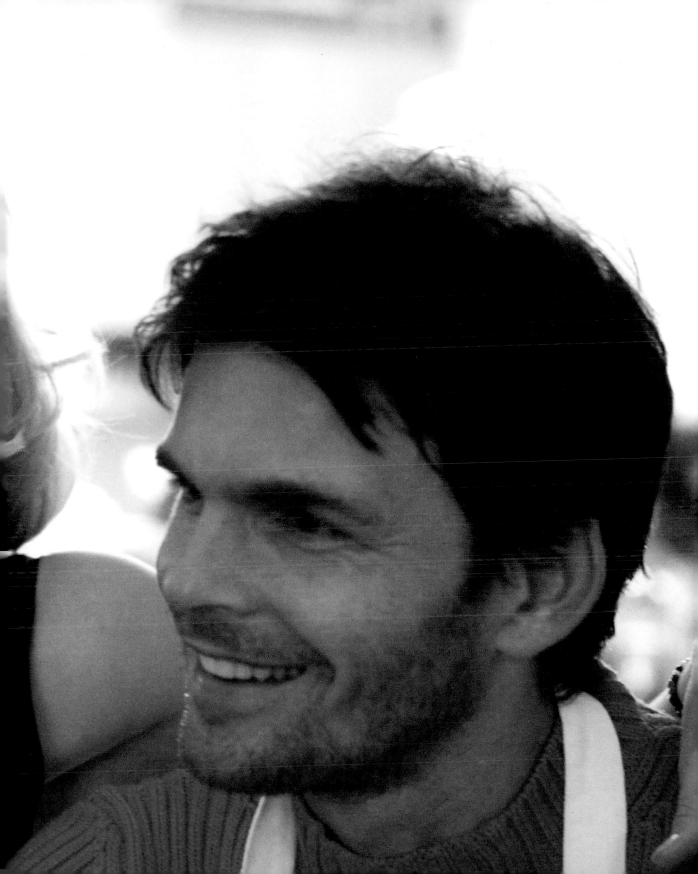

White Sangria

SERVES 4

Without being sweet and without losing the character of the wine, this concoction is ideal for the summer (or when you want to pretend that it's summer). Use a nice dry wine, which will have plenty of sweetness in the essence, and really fresh, ripe, chilled fruit, cut into small pieces. Assuming all the fruit is organic, keep the peel on the citrus fruits; the slightly bitter rind is actually tasty to chew, especially after soaking in the wine.

> This is best made a few hours in advance and chilled. We prefer to serve this in a large wine glass (and with a spoon). When in season, try using apple mint—a sweet and mild variety you can find at a greenmarket. —MK

1 bottle dry Sauvignon Blanc (we prefer a grassy, gooseberry-laden New Zealand variety)
4 cups ice cubes
1 peach, pitted and chopped
1 cup chopped pineapple
1 green apple, cored and chopped
1 orange, sliced, seeds removed, and chopped
1 lime, sliced and chopped
2 to 3 tablespoons agave nectar
2 tablespoons lemon juice
2 to 3 sprigs fresh mint

In a large pitcher, add all the ingredients except the mint and stir well. If not serving right away, keep the sangria chilled in the refrigerator. Garnish each glass with fresh mint.

Spiced Pear Sake-Tini

SERVES 4

Try to use a really sweet, rich pear juice, which is best from very ripe fruit.

When our bartender Joey first made
this for me, it was like drinking the most comforting,
fall weather dessert. —SM

3 cups fresh pear juice

1 cup sake

2 tablespoons agave nectar

Splash of fresh ginger juice

Pinch of ground cinnamon

In a martini shaker, pour all the ingredients over ice and shake or stir very well to chill. Strain and pour into martini glasses.

Thai Lemonade

SERVES 6 TO 8

Lemonade is the one drink that everyone seems to love. Thai basil works nicely in this with mint—you can use either or both. And, of course, feel free to add a splash of sake and champagne if you want a real cocktail!

1 cup lemon juice

$^1/_4$ cup lime juice

$^1/_2$ cup agave nectar

4 cups filtered water

2 tablespoons lemongrass juice

Pinch of cayenne pepper

1 small handful Thai basil leaves and/or mint leaves

In a large pitcher, mix all ingredients with a lot of ice and chill.

Frozen Grape Champagne

SERVES 6 TO 8

We know we preach that *seeded* grapes (and other fruit) are always preferable to *seedless*, which are hybridized. Seeded grapes would be fine in this recipe as long as you blend them thoroughly and don't mind a bit of grittiness. However, in this case, the ones without the seeds make a much more texturally pleasant drink. Just be sure to make it immediately before serving, as the blended grapes begin to turn color after a little while.

> **Grapes with grapes . . . it seems so obvious that when we first thought of it, we wondered why we'd never seen it anywhere before.** —SM

1 large bunch green grapes, preferably seedless, pulled from stems and frozen solid
2 to 3 tablespoons lemon juice
1 full bottle champagne or sparkling wine

In a blender, puree the frozen grapes with the lemon juice and about half of the champagne. You may need to do this in batches if it all won't fit in your blender. Add the remaining champagne, pulse the blender just to combine, and serve immediately in flutes.

Sake Colada

SERVES 4

This drink is the happier variation of the Piña Colada on page 70.

2 cups chopped pineapple

1/2 cup coconut meat

1/2 cup coconut water

1/4 cup agave nectar

1 tablespoon lime juice

1 teaspoon vanilla extract

2 cups ice

3/4 cups sake

pinch sea salt

In a blender, puree all the ingredients and serve immediately.

Pineapple Lemongrass-Tini

SERVES 4 TO 6

Pineapple and lemongrass naturally complement each other. To juice the lemongrass, peel away the outer husk, chop the stalk into a few pieces, and run it through the juicer with the pineapple.

2 cups pineapple juice

1/2 thin stalk lemongrass, juiced

1/4 cup lime juice

1/2 cup sake

1/4 cup champagne or sparkling wine

In a martini shaker, pour all the ingredients except champagne over ice and shake or stir very well to chill. Strain and pour into martini glasses. Top with champagne.

Plum-Passion Fruit Long Island Iced Tea

SERVES 4

Plum–passion fruit tea and sake seem to be made for each other in this delicious cocktail. Although the combination of flavors may seem exotic, it is quite balanced and subtle.
We use an organic plum and passion fruit–flavored tea, although most fruity or berry-
based teas will work very well here.

1 $^1/_2$ cups steeped and chilled plum–passion fruit tea
1 cup sake
$^1/_2$ cup lime juice
$^1/_4$ cup agave nectar
Lemon or lime wedges for garnish

In a large pitcher, combine the tea, sake, lime juice, and agave nectar and stir well. Pour
into cocktail glasses or tall glasses full of ice and garnish with lemon or lime wedges.

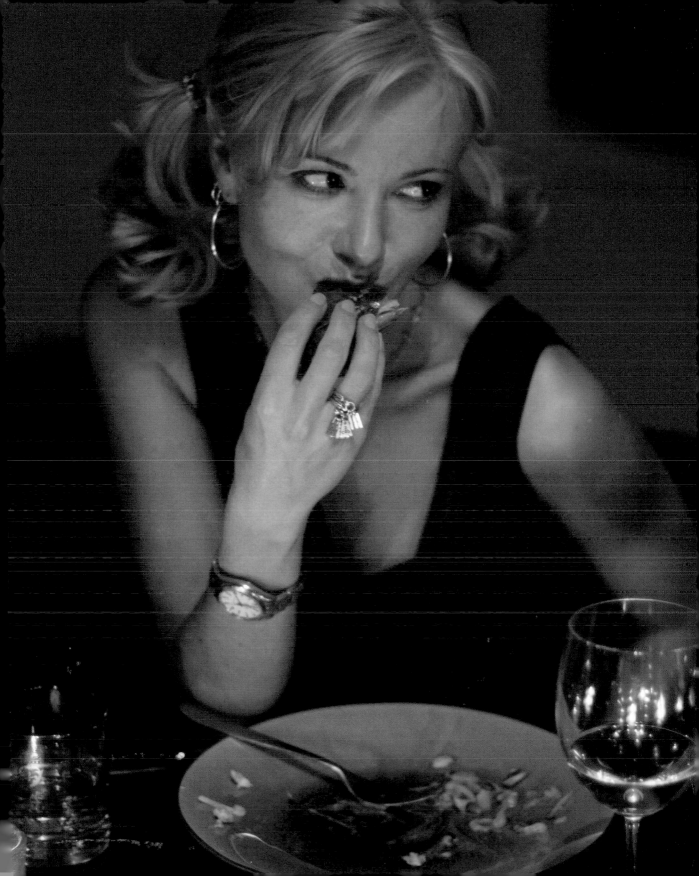

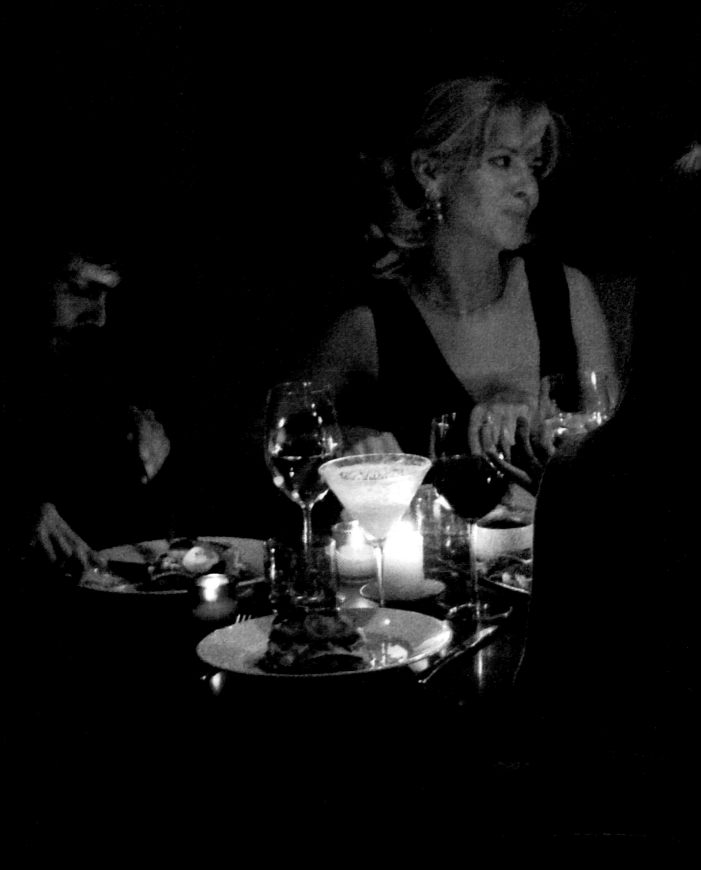

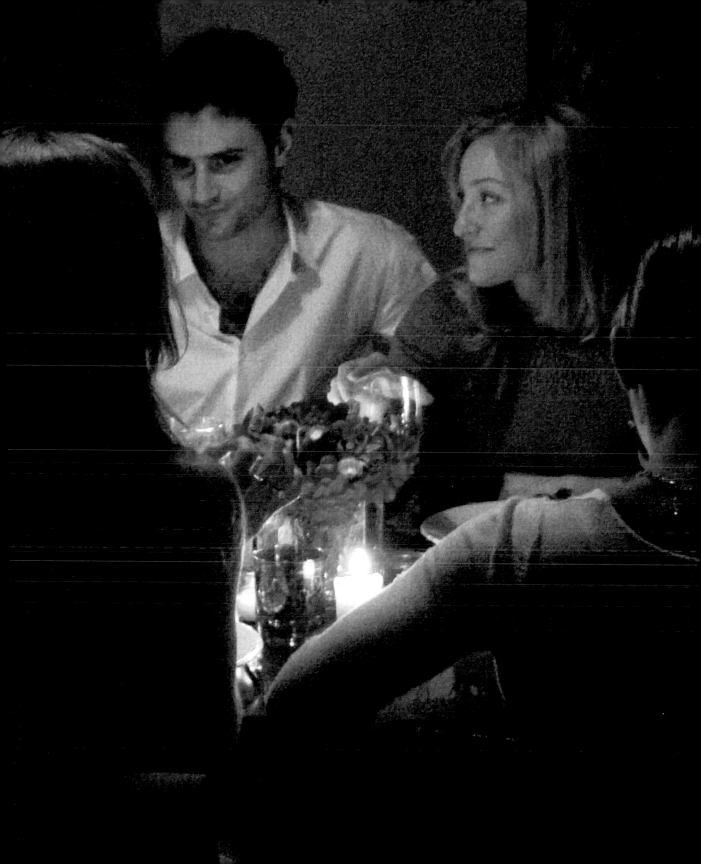

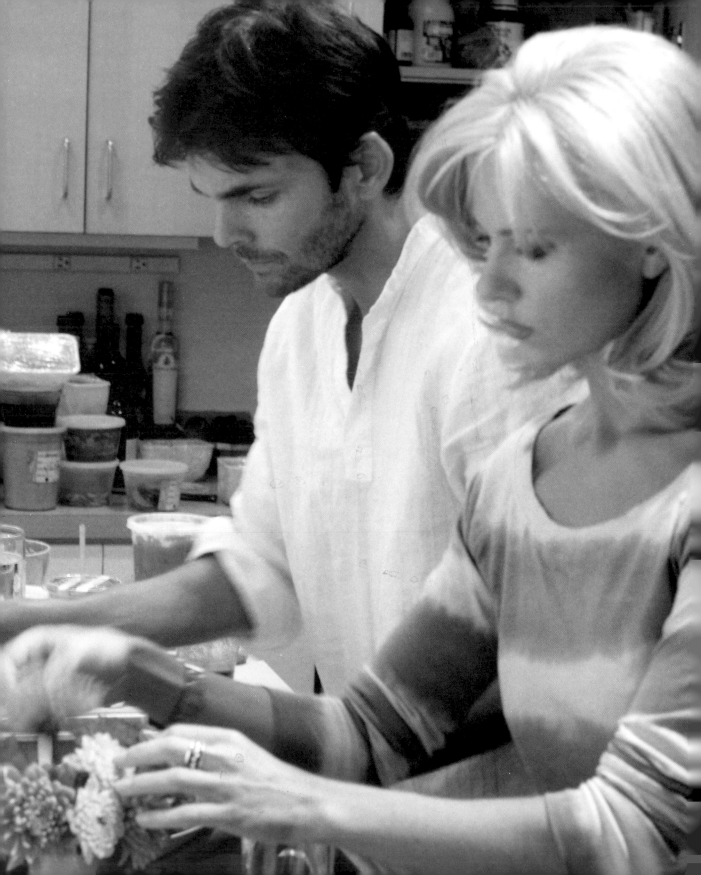

AFTERWORD
THE REAL WORLD

While we truly believe that raw foods can change your life, we also don't feel that it should necessarily *rule* your life. Changing your eating habits does not mean that you need to stop shaving your armpits and start listening to more folk music. Nor does it mean that you need to stop going out with your meat-eating friends so that you can attend weekly raw food potlucks . . . unless you want to do all those things and they make you happy! There is certainly much support to be gained through meeting other people participating in the raw foods lifestyle, and networking within the community can be very valuable, encouraging, and satisfying.

Having signed up for tons of raw food newsletters, we've heard about and been invited to various events, from community sing-alongs to raw foodist hugathons. We were once very tempted to go to a 'Raw Chocolate Aphrodisiac Party,' which sounded intriguing, except I was too scared! I had visions of getting sucked into some kind of creepy orgy with hemp clothing flying off everywhere and lots of itchy dreadlocks.   —SM

As with many things in life, when it comes to diet, we think it does not need to be taken all *too* seriously. We hope that many of you will gain some knowledge from this book about incorporating more raw foods into your lifestyle. For others, you may be inspired to change your habits entirely, as we did. You may in fact take it *very* seriously if you have acute health issues or know someone who is or has been ill and healed themselves with raw foods and a natural lifestyle. There are countless such stories, and we meet people all the time who tell us their personal healing stories resulting from their change to raw foods. It is endlessly inspiring.

However, it's easy to get very caught up, overwhelmed, and maybe even discouraged while making a change that can sometimes require a lot of effort and also impacts our working days, relationships, and social lives. Going out with friends or accepting a dinner invitation at someone's house and then trying to explain your "peculiar" eating habits can become challenging and even stressful. If you start immersing yourself in all things raw and plowing through books and research, you may get a bit overzealous and start worrying your family. You may even decide (as we did) to embark on detoxifying cleanses or fasts. Furthermore, it is not uncommon to experience some slightly *odd* symptoms that could cause a bit of alarm. This chapter focuses on those areas of the raw food world not directly related to recipes and food preparation, but that are a very real and relevant part of this lifestyle.

Raw Foods and the Rest of the World

We believe it's important to keep in mind that this whole process should be *fun*, and we think that the best approach is to be open minded. Remember, this is not a temporary diet, or a strict Atkins-like regimen (you can imagine how we feel about the Atkins diet)—where you can disrupt the whole program with a bite of bread and have to start all over again. So rather than holding ourselves to the strictest standards with this way of eating, we feel reasonably comfortable compromising here and there.

We are not the type to go into a restaurant and demand something special that's not on the menu, or to ask for a plate of sliced raw vegetables (particularly if it's a good restaurant). Nor do we want to make our diet the topic of every conversation. When we first started eating this way, and before we were fully "out of the closet," we were occasionally invited out to dinner with friends, where we would attempt to order vegetarian and simply do the best we could, while trying to at least enjoy any deviation from our normal raw food consumption. We did not want to make a big thing of it. It should also be noted that the dinner table is generally not the best venue for explaining to your company the philosophy behind your new lifestyle. People don't really want to hear about hormones and antibiotics, mad cow, or the putrefication and clogging going on in their intestines *while* they are chewing on their steak.

> At times, I feel very outspoken and want to run around spreading knowledge that I truly believe in my heart can make people healthier and happier. Yet much of the time, I keep to myself out of respect for people's ways, for traditions, and for the sake of not wanting to offend anyone. But it can be hard. I feel so much better and happier living this way, that I want the people that I care about to be able to feel this way, too! —SM

If you've ever worked in a traditional kitchen or restaurant, if you love restaurants and food and dine out regularly, hang out in the food world, or just have one of those families where everything seems to revolve around traditional cooking—then you might be well aware of the ridicule and often condescension thrown in the direction of vegetarians and vegans. We have both lived in that world for a long time and were therefore fully prepared for the assault of jokes, mockery, and even hostility that would come our way. It's important to have a sense of humor, but while we can be easy-going and appreciate it, at the end of the day, we still hold fast to our views.

Consider Anthony Bourdain, the cigarette-smoking, heavy drinking, swaggering chef/food journalist, who makes no bones (pardon the pun) about his disdain for vegetarians and vegans. In his best selling book, *Kitchen Confidential,* he calls vegans "the Hezbollah of vegetarians" (okay, that's funny) and in a more recent article said that raw foodists espouse "a philosophy so extreme as to make ordinary vegans look like libertines." In this same article he claims that Roxanne Klein and Charlie Trotter's book, *Raw,* is a "poke in the eye to the entire culinary profession." So now you see what we mean about the hostility and ridicule! In this same article Bourdain concludes, "At a time in history when Americans have reasons to turn away from this fabulously diverse and marvelous planet, the authors have made willful avoidance and abstinence a more attractive option. I admire their skills. But I fear for the planet."

That's an interesting stand to take. Fresh fruits and vegetables *are* really scary. Although what about the opposite viewpoint?

"Nothing will benefit human health and increase the chances for survival of life on Earth as much as the evolution to a vegetarian diet."

—ALBERT EINSTEIN (a vegetarian himself, obviously)

Anthony Bourdain or Albert Einstein? Hmmmm.

If I ever needed guidance on how to skin a rabbit or whip up a tasty dish of blood sausage, I'd seek out Tony's expertise. But when it comes to matters such as the fate of our earth, I'll give more weight to Einstein's words. I love Bourdain's books and I read most every article he writes. He's hilarious and at least honest about his views. I think he would be a fabulous and fascinating companion on an exotic food trip (not that he would go with me). I went to Spain recently where I ate everything offered to me during a particularly amazing twenty-six course tasting menu, including such things as bacon-wrapped banana, foie gras, and pigeon, and I thoroughly appreciated the flavors of every bite. I think I'm open minded

We do understand that many people may not agree with what we express about food. Choosing what to eat and feeding others are very personal processes and intertwined with the notion of taking care of ourselves and other people, particularly our loved ones. There are centuries of tradition related to various preparations of meat, artisanal cheeses, and cooking of all sorts of foods—much of which it may seem we have just flippantly dismissed as "toxic." We agree that there is something very sad about the rejection of much of this history and tradition. Further, it is not our intention to pass judgment on the way some people eat. Ideally, we'd rather simply focus on the benefits of raw plant foods, without demonizing meat, dairy, and all things cooked. But it's hard to fully convey our passion for this way of eating without illustrating what we've learned. This is especially true when we believe the information to be very accurate and portentous about the way much of the country eats today (and therefore we *do* think that commercial junk food and specifically mass-produced meat and dairy could always use some bashing!)

One of the more challenging aspects of shifting to raw foods and fully embracing the philosophy is how difficult it becomes to watch people you care about not taking care of themselves in the way that we might now wish that they would. But by the same token, it's also extremely rewarding when we're able to have a positive impact on the people around us, without even really trying!

When we were building Pure Food and Wine, our contractor and friend Russell liked to make fun of the food we were serving. Pretty soon though, he began eating it as we began testing recipes in the new kitchen. Then he had a wheatgrass shot one day and began drinking green juice the next. Russell

While it's not that hard to imagine making the transition to raw foods when working in or around a place like our restaurant and juice bar it can be a great deal more challenging in other environments. If you live in a big city like New York, or Los Angeles especially, where raw foods are very popular, it is far easier than if you live, say, in the rural areas of North Dakota, where there probably aren't too many organic co-op markets to choose from! Online sources are very handy for stocking up if you live in a remote location (see Sources, page 357). You can even order produce online, although this does not really flow with the idea of eating locally. If there's nothing available in your immediate area, however, it's a good option to keep in mind.

We were fortunate in our early stages to have friends who could guide us and also to live in an area where it was possible to buy fresh nut milks only a few blocks from our home. The further along we progressed, the easier it became to develop strategies for when we might be traveling or otherwise away from home. So many books we've read have quite seriously suggested taking a Vita-Mix with you when you travel. We presume that the majority of our readers wouldn't want to lug an expensive and *very* heavy blender through security and baggage check at the airport (they would probably pull it apart and confiscate the blade, anyway!). Nor is it easy to imagine setting it up in your hotel room, or washing the blender cup (where—in the bathtub?). Who has time for that sort of thing when traveling, particularly if visiting somewhere beautiful with fresh food available!

Depending on where we are going and how long we'll be there, we generally just try to bring snacks like spiced nuts, some dried fruits or raw cookies, and whatever fruit we can carry for the commute. Manna bread with almond butter is always a nice thing to bring as well. Otherwise, we just rely on what we can find wherever we are going. We also try to keep in mind that being hungry is not the end of the world. In fact, there is abundant research about how fasting for various durations is actually extremely healthy and promotes longevity.

Open Letter:
From Mad Cows to Madmen

This is to inform you that we are pissed as hell.

First you lock us up in deplorable living conditions. Then you pump us full of antibiotics so we don't become ill from those conditions. And then you give us steroids to make us bigger and fatter—all so you can become bigger and fatter.

This "mad cow" thing is the final straw. It's not enough that you made us—who were born vegans—into carnivorous cannibals by grinding up bones and body parts of our brothers and cousins and turning them into "meal." Now you blame us for a terminal disease that has struck down mere hundreds of you to date.

Apologies if you find that rather unsympathetic, but a lot more of us have died from the disease than you even suspect. Try about 1,000 of us per week back at the height of the first epidemic in 1993, and hundreds of thousands destroyed during the second epidemic in 2001. (And throughout the decades, millions of us have been slaughtered for Happy Meals—it says so right on the sign).

Allow us to tell you the truth about mad cow disease. It's a deviation of a naturally occurring, rare neurological disorder that strikes both humans and animals, vegetarians and meat-eaters alike. In humans, it's called Creutzfeldt-Jakob Disease (CJD) and is caused by prions that can't be killed by cooking or freezing. Neither bacteria nor virus, a prion is a vicious little protein that lives on the surface of the cell. Yet it can become disease-producing and replicate without having DNA, so scientists are still trying to understand what *that's* all about. These renegade prions only live in the central nervous system (brain and spinal cord), not tissue or bone, and they destroy it pretty rapidly. A rapid onset of the three D's—debilitation, degeneration, and dementia—leads to a fourth one, death. But consider this: your chances of coming down with classic CJD, which strikes 1 in 1 million per year, are about the same as winning the lottery, and as random (except here you pray for the pleasure of losing).

In us, prion disease is called bovine spongiform encephalopathy (BSE). When it spreads from us to a human—because you inadvertently ate parts of an infected animal's nervous system, usually found in ground beef—it's called variant Creutzfeldt-Jakob Disease, or vCJD. Currently, vCJD can be possibly contracted from cows in any of thirty-three host countries to date (in addition to the diaspora of its exportation). Incubation time is unknown. Treatment is unavailable. Your odds are anybody's guess. It's hardly a roulette game worth playing.

But while there are plenty of questions left to be answered about both CJD and vCJD, a ready solution presents itself. Stop eating us. It's like abstinence. You can't get pregnant if you don't have sex. Or Nancy Reagan's policy: Just say no. You can't become an addict if you don't do the drug. We guarantee, we'll all be a whole lot happier.

When I went to Spain recently, I left for the long commute with nothing but a bottle of water. I was delayed at the airport and then missed my connection as well. It ultimately took about 20 hours before I was in my hotel room. During that time, I may have felt hungry a few times, but it didn't last very long and I felt good. Fasting when the only thing around is airplane food and airport junk food is *not* hard at all—as it certainly does not feel like any kind of sacrifice. I also knew that I'd be taken to all kinds of amazing restaurants during my trip and tasting lots of things not raw and not vegan, so it was nice to give my system a break before the onslaught. I could have very easily brought plenty of raw snacks with me, but what for? I didn't feel I really needed them.   —SM

When I've traveled for business since going raw, Sarma would often pack snacks for me or I would bring cut fruit in containers for the flight. I've found that no matter where I've gone, it's never really that hard to find fruit, including my favorite, avocados. It's very easy at a restaurant to ask for a sliced avocado with a salad, or even to buy them at a store and eat them plain (this is actually my favorite way). Avocados, when ripe and eaten alone, are an amazingly luscious and satisfying food.   —MK

One of the things you might notice after going raw for long enough is that your body actually becomes more accepting of other foods. We've met so many people who speak about having been 100 percent raw for a certain number of years, which is great. We eat almost 100 percent raw (aside from the occasional bit of cocoa or maple or other ingredient) all of the time in our everyday lives. But, we both love restaurants and traveling, and for the sake of enjoying these experiences we are comfortable enough eating small amounts of other foods on occasion. When your systems are clean and running efficiently, whatever foods you eat, whether raw or cooked, will be digested that much more easily. If your body has been cleansed with raw foods, the occasional moderate detour off the raw food wagon should not cause too much trouble.

Detox and Our Adventures in Cleansing

A significant component of a shift to raw foods is detoxification and cleansing—both increasingly often-heard buzzwords in the media these days. So far we have been gloating about the various ways in which we have felt so much *better* living this lifestyle, but there were times throughout our transition that we were detoxifying and felt a bit less than amazing. Further, since we came across this new lifestyle during a time when we did not have demanding schedules, we found we had ample time to get fascinated by and wrapped up in all kinds of cleansing experimentation. We went to seminars, and we listened to raw food gurus and healers. We bought their products, took their advice, and enthusiastically tried various regimens to purify ourselves (we hoped) and had some interesting experiences along the way. We followed herbal fasts, discovered the often bizarre world of colonics, and even tried to rid our bodies of unwanted gallstones by following an extreme regimen that required us to ingest all sorts of unpleasant things and excrete things beyond unpleasant. Stay tuned!

Detox

Detoxification refers to your body literally purging toxins, presumably accumulated during years of less-than-thoughtful consumption of food and drink, smoking and taking drugs (prescribed or otherwise), and everyday pollution from the environment and household products.

A transition to a primarily all raw diet can be smooth and painless, or it can get a bit uncomfortable and even strange at times, generally depending on the prior state of your digestive health and the pace at which you incorporate raw foods into your diet. It can be very much like giving up coffee: if you drink ten cups a day, and then try to quit overnight, your body will rebel and express it through *pain*, primarily headaches in this case. However, if you slowly decrease to 9 cups, then 8, then 7, your system can gradually and smoothly adjust. With raw foods, it can be similar and you might experience some degree of discomfort as your body rids itself of these various accumulated toxins. For most people, this is very minimal—perhaps a few days of feeling bloated, a bit headachy, or simply tired. This is a normal part of the adjustment process, but very important to be aware of, as you might give up right away if you don't instantly feel better, thinking it's not right for you.

If you plow through books on raw food the way we did, you can easily get caught up in it. The list of possible symptoms of "detox" is so all-inclusive, from headaches to fever to skin rashes, that every random twitch or itch becomes suspect. For us it got a bit out of hand such that for any little bump or blemish we noticed, we'd just look at each other and say, "DETOX!!" Theoretically, the more "toxic" you were to begin with and the more suddenly you make the change, the more frequent and severe your body's reponse will be. While we made the change very abruptly, we were also fortunately used to eating large salads and lots of fresh fruits, especially in the summertime, so overall, what we experienced was relatively mild, although often *interesting*.

> My stomach felt bloated on and off for a number of days, and I would at times feel quite lethargic. I began losing weight right away as well. Then periodically, Sarma or I would have an extremely runny nose, but for a very short duration— just a couple of hours. Like a flash flood. It was funny, and somewhat fascinating. All these oddities did indeed seem to be some kind of expression of our bodies expelling something.   —MK

In his book, *The Sunfood Diet Success System*, David Wolfe includes a chapter that very rationally and helpfully describes the process of detoxification. He claims that what we eat either thickens our blood (cooked and heavy foods) or thins our blood (raw foods), and that as our blood becomes thinner than our lymph fluids, the accumulated toxins in those fluids are able to be released into the blood, and from there filtered out as wastes. While it may not always be comfortable, keep in mind that this detoxification is a good thing, and will always pass. Wolfe also recommends ways in which to speed up or slow down detoxification: essentially, eating only fruit and vegetable juices speed ups detox, while adding heavier foods such as avocados and oils, or even cooked foods such as steamed vegetables, slows it down a bit.

Adventures in Cleansing

As you will quickly learn, if you leap feet first into the world of raw food, it's not always just about the food you eat on a daily basis. While eating raw foods will cleanse your system over a period of time, there are ways to speed up the process, if you feel you want to go down that road! In the raw food community, it's easy to be bombarded with information about cleansing your system through various programs of fasting, with or without various herbs and supplements and/or colonics. Many books are full of cleansing advice, and the raw food stores we visited were very oriented towards cleanses and all the related products and supplies. It can be very easy to get caught up in all of it, as we certainly did.

To clean your colon or not to clean your colon? That is a hotly debated subject among raw foodists and others. Some say that "colon hydrotherapy" is essential for ridding your body of toxins and the accumulated "mucoid plaque" in your intestines. Others say that it's an unnatural invasion of sorts, and that we should let our bodies cleanse themselves naturally by letting the clean, fiber-rich foods we eat sweep out the impurities, without also pulling out the good intestinal "flora" that a colonic drains out. Nevertheless, we had to try it!

While it seems now that every new fancy spa is offering colonics (it's well-known to be increasingly popular for Hollywood stars to go for colonics before having to walk down the red carpet in those tight dresses) we somehow ended up finding our way to one of the more bizarre establishments. First-time visitors are made to watch a truly gory twenty-minute video that should be titled, "Everything You *Never Ever* Wanted to Know About Your Colon." The video looked like it was made in the seventies—also, incidentally, the last time the place had been redecorated.

Once I got over the weirdness of it all, I sort of got into the whole colonics thing for a while, and liked that feeling of emptiness immediately following each session. Naturally, I signed up for the ten session program complete with herbs, enzymes, and probiotic supplements after being convinced that the 'black, tar-like' buildup in my colon would be expelled, lightening my intestines (and forever flattening my lower belly). The thing is, no 'black tar-like' buildup was ever seen exiting my colon, and I was subsequently told that I must not have had any, due to my relatively healthy lifelong diet including lots of fruits and vegetables. You would think this would be good news, but somehow I was disappointed.   —SM

The herbal intestinal cleanse combined with colonics was a walk in the park compared to the grueling 14-day "gallstone cleanse" that we bravely attempted. There are many variations on this cleanse, but of course we came across the most complicated version of all. Aside from all the weirdness we were ingesting, we had to soak flannel in castor oil and plastic wrap it to our bodies for an hour or so each day, presumably to soften the stones. And this was only part of the fun. Believe it or not, we're leaving out some of the gorier details! But after the climactic consumption of a full cup of olive oil (with a little lemon juice on the side), we both were ridiculously ecstatic to then "pass" a whole bunch of gallstones. Or so we thought. While the process was rough, at least (we told each other) all those stones were not in our bodies anymore. So we felt pretty good about that until a few weeks later when we came across an article in a health magazine by Dr. Andrew Weil, the very popular author of many books related to health and alternative medicine, about various cleansing programs. He mentioned that he suspected that the gallstones excreted after this increasingly popular cleanse, might in fact really be just the coagulated olive oil and lemon juice and nothing more. We asked a raw M.D. that we know, and he thought this claim might be possible. We are still *very* curious to know the truth!

At this point, we'll still go for the occasional colonic, but we gave up quickly on the harsh cleanses, especially the ones that start to feel like bizarre forms of torture with each passing day. But we have met *many* people who have had much success with both of these types of programs. And, as always, we'll remain open minded about these and other practices related to cleansing and detoxifying (Sarma especially!).   —MK

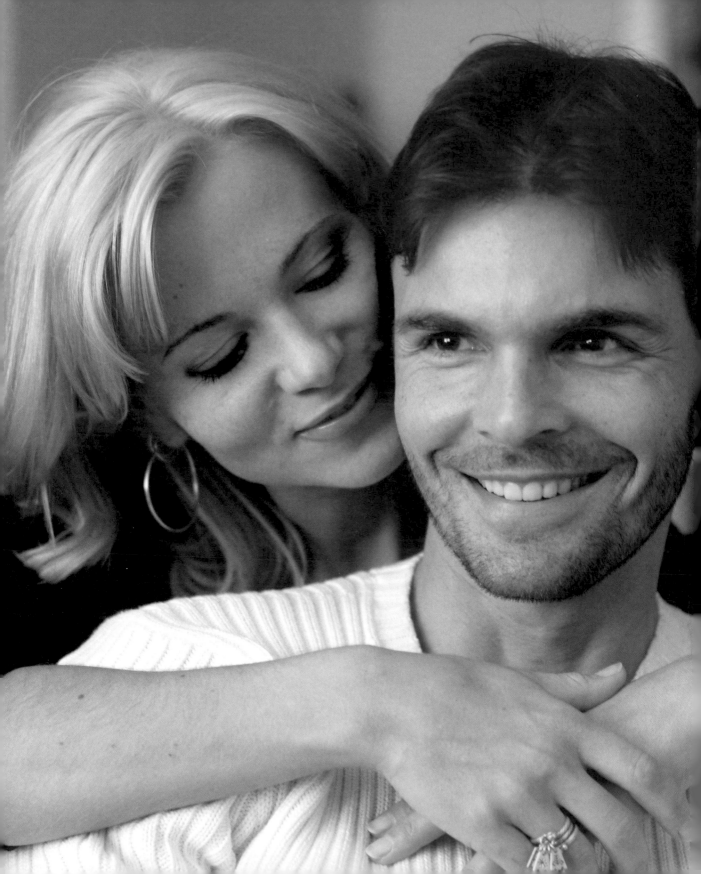

It's Not Just the Food You Eat

Once you open your eyes and become acutely aware of the importance of what you put *in* your body for fuel (not to mention what comes out!), it is hard not to begin examining all of the things around you as well. What is in those lotions we rub all over our skin? What is that harsh smell we're breathing in as we mop the floor? *And why is there a skull and crossbones on the label?* From there, we can't help thinking differently about the garbage we create, the useless products we buy and the materials they are made of, the paint on our walls, the fibers and dyes of the clothes we wear and the sheets we sleep on, and so forth. Eating uncooked, unprocessed, natural foods can be only the beginning!

When we came back to New York City after our first few weeks on raw food in Maine, we felt unusually aware of how unclean the streets and the air felt. Although we had both lived in the city for over ten years, it was the first time that we really became fixated on the pollution and the dirtiness of the air. We're certainly not going to leave New York any time soon, but it was interesting how quickly our perceptions about our environment were changing. It was as if living clean on the inside was making us want to live clean in so many other ways as well!

As we continued our research and reading about raw foods, we also began to further appreciate the importance of not just eating organically, but of living organically, too—as much as possible. Just as it makes sense to shun foods treated with pesticides or containing chemicals, it also makes sense to avoid inhaling or absorbing those substances. One by one we began replacing things in our home such as laundry detergents, cleaning supplies, shampoo, toothpaste, soaps, and lotions, with organic versions. We started buying only the recycled, unbleached brands of paper towels and recycled trash bags. We even put our cats on a raw, organic diet! Reading about hemp products is very compelling, and we started buying some hemp things, including our favorite: a hemp shower curtain. Think about all of those thick, plastic shower curtains that everyone buys, that end up clogging a landfill somewhere!

I read somewhere an estimate that women, on average, consume about 4 pounds of lipstick in their lifetime. It makes sense if you think about it—where does all that constantly reapplied lipstick go? Some on coffee cups or on napkins (and

You Are What You Wear

Have you noticed the increasing popularity of using the patch as a delivery system for prescription and over-the-counter medications? These are, in fact, more efficient, because the drugs get delivered directly into your bloodstream instead of first being digested and absorbed through the stomach lining. It's convenient and it works.

So what happens when you slather your body with an artificially scented, chemically preserved lotion made with ingredients that may be toxic and are completely unregulated by the FDA or anyone else? It goes into your blood. Same for face and eye creams, body washes, soap, scents, self-tanners, sunscreens, and cosmetics. Some Victorian women used arsenic solutions to whiten their faces that caused them to sicken and die. Did you ever notice the labels of some skin products warn that they should not be ingested under any circumstances?

Cosmetic and skin care manufacturers can use any ingredients they want and are not required to do safety testing—in fact, they are not even required to fully disclose all of the ingredients on the label, under the guise of protecting their formulas from competition. The European Union has banned hundreds of ingredients from personal care products in contrast to just a small handful banned by the FDA. For an extremely compelling and comprehensive review of the dangers in cosmetics and skin care, we encourage you to check out www.beautytruth.net, researched and put together by a makeup artist to the fashion industry who has personally experienced the havoc that these toxins can wreak. As the title suggests, her site reveals the fallacies behind cosmetic and skin care labels and outlines the ingredients we should avoid.

There's something very liberating about minimizing the amount of clutter in your bathroom medicine cabinet. We both now regularly use olive oil or coconut butter—the same that we use in our food—in place of body lotion, face cream, and bath oil. Coconut butter also makes an excellent stand-in for shaving cream and is a tasty lip balm! For many of the products that we buy, a good general guideline when checking the ingredients is to look for only things that you wouldn't mind eating: Now our trips to those huge, fluorescently lit drugstores are very rare, and when we do go in, we find ourselves somewhat in awe of all the *crap* they sell. It's a bit like looking at the world through a new set of lenses.

For anyone serious about raw foods, there is a natural
evolution that occurs, that will take you on a journey. That
journey will open your eyes to the beauty of our planet and
give you a reason to care more about it, to treat it with less
abandon, to love all animals, and eventually have trouble
understanding why things have evolved the way they have.
These discoveries were all quite shocking, especially for a
couple of ex-carnivore chefs.   —MK

Closing Thoughts

Raw food and the lifestyle associated with it are so compelling and complex that we will be forever learning and growing. Already, it seems that we have discovered some of the magic that life offers. When I find something that makes me happy, gives me health and vitality, or simply amuses me, I will often search for a deeper meaning within that and find other layers of positive elements that I work into my life. Such was the case with our raw food experience. You will have your own journey and will make decisions based on your own experiences; the events of our own transition were rapid and all consuming— and definitely worth sharing. Still, there is more—much more— and we will continue to search and experiment. We hope to have the opportunity to pass those lessons along and do whatever we can to provide more people with the joy that this movement has brought to us. —MK

I had always thought that Matthew and I were extremely healthy people. Cooking, restaurants, and good food have long been passions for both of us. If someone had told me only a few years ago that I would become a vegetarian, eating exclusively *raw* plant foods on a daily basis, waking up without my coffee, and passing through the afternoons without Diet Coke, I would have assumed that person was smoking crack. But I also never before knew what it felt like to experience life the way that we do now. I feel like I never *really* tasted things the way I do now and never before marveled at the intricate and fascinating shapes of all the varieties of fruits and vegetables available to us. And I certainly never felt as nourished, inspired, excited, and gratified by food as I do today. It's very empowering to know that our personal choices, as individuals, can so dramatically affect the future of our own health and quality of life, and that those same choices, collectively, could move markets, shift tides, and improve the quality of life on earth for future generations. It may sound overly dramatic, but the whole framework through which I view the world has changed. Life is beautiful. Eat raw and live long. —SM

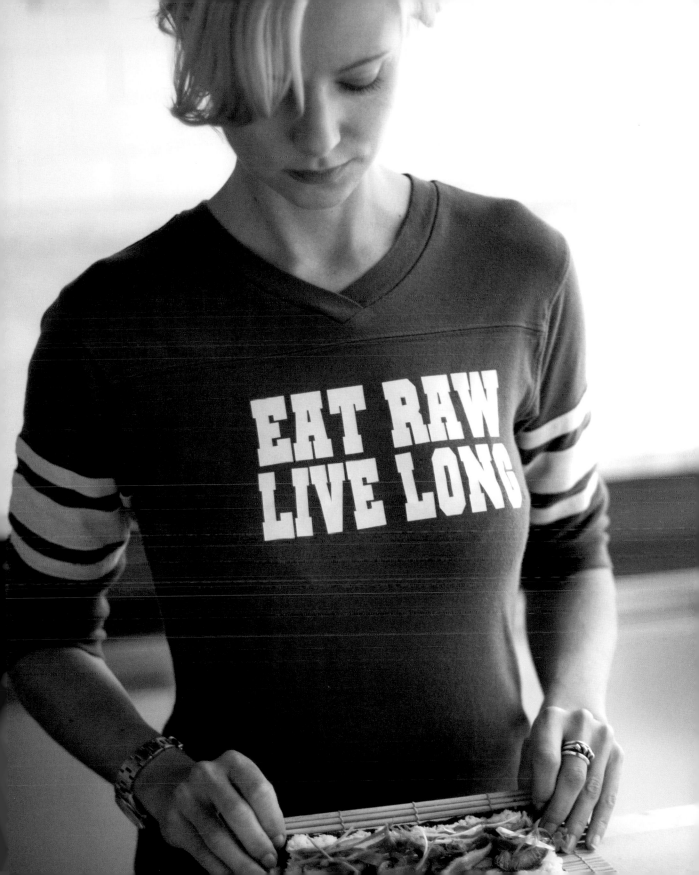

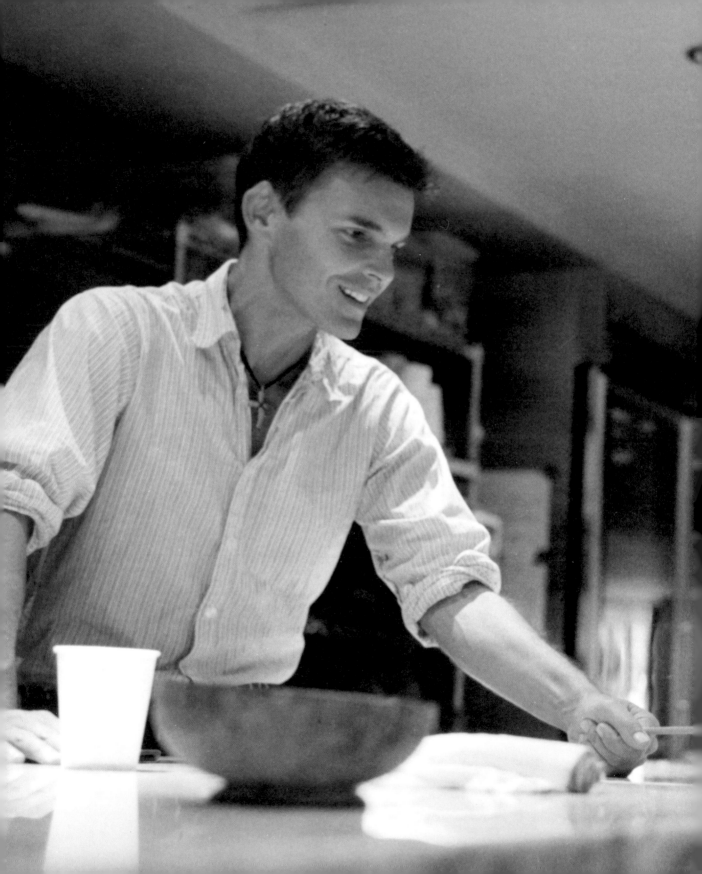

SOURCES

It all seems backward, and in fact, it is: you'll often need to search far and wide to find ingredients that are natural and unadulterated, while those that are processed and refined beyond recognition are easily located practically at our doorsteps. Fortunately, there is a growing contingency of dedicated suppliers who work hard to bring us the best in natural, organic, healthful products. We spend a great deal of time searching for these suppliers and their companies. Due to the very specialized market in which many of these products are sold, we find that many of them carry limited, but very high quality, products.

To that end, we are creating a source of our own that will supply most everything one would need to get started and maintain a raw, organic lifestyle, as well as other great products, ongoing advice, books, kitchen equipment, discussion, and news. Most of the products listed below and many others will be available at oneluckyduck.com. The link to this website and to information about our other projects can also be found at rawfoodrealworld.com.

Most of the more common ingredients (nuts, seeds) as well as harder to find ingredients—those specific to raw foods as well as a few of the more obscure seasonings that we have used in recipes in this book—are listed below.

Agave Nectar: This sweetener can be found at many health food stores and raw food outlets. If your local health food store does not carry it, you may want to ask them to do so. Online, try shopnatural.com or oneluckyduck.com.

Avocado Oil: Elysian Isle is the brand that we use, and the avocado-lime variety is our favorite. You can buy it directly from them at elysianisle.com.

Bee Pollen: Every health food store generally carries bee pollen, but for the best quality, try oneluckyduck.com, rawfood.com or highvibe.com.

Blue-Green Algae: For Crystal Manna, our favorite, go to oneluckyduck.com or ancientsuninc.com.

Cacao Beans: For raw cacao beans, or nibs (sold in broken pieces, which is generally just fine), go to oneluckyduck.com or rawfood.com.

Carob Powder: It's not always easy to find raw carob powder and there are many fla-vor variations. For the best quality, try highvibe.com or oneluckyduck.com.

Chunky Chat Masala: Available at Indian grocery stores and kalustyans.com.

Cocoa Powder: Green & Black's, made in the United Kingdom, is our favorite brand of organic cocoa. You can find it at some health food stores, at oneluckyduck.com, or chocosphere.com (which also carries Dagoba, another good brand).

Coconuts, Young Thai: These are becoming increasingly easy to find at whole foods and health food stores, and are available at Asian markets. Purchasing online is expensive because of the high cost of shipping, but they are available at young coconuts.com.

Coconut Butter/Oil: The very best kind we've ever come across is called Virgin Oil de Coco-Crème and you can find it at oneluckyduck.com and highvibe.com. Always be sure to smell it before using. The flavor should be fresh and coconutty or very neutral. If it has a toasted flavor or just smells off, it may have gone rancid or is just an inferior product and could adversely affect the taste of whatever you use it in.

Date Sugar: This can be used in place of maple sugar and is available at many health food stores or at shopnatural.com or diamondorganics.com.

Dried Fruits: It's not always easy to find organic, unsulphured dried fruits, and very often dried fruits have been sweetened with sugar, so check carefully before you buy. Try organicfruitsandnuts.com or highvibe.com for a reliable source for good quality dried fruits.

E3-Live: You can find this amazing frozen liquid algae in the freezers of some health food stores, or it can be ordered to ship frozen online at E3live.com. We will also carry many E3live products at our own site.

Galangal, Fresh: You can usually find this at Asian markets. If you can't, fresh ginger is a better substitute than dried galangal in most cases.

Grains and Seeds: Most grains are available at health food stores, but try diamondorganics.com to find buckwheat groats, quinoa, flaxseeds, and others.

Hemp Protein: Available at freshhempfoods.com and oneluckyduck.com

Hemp Seeds: Available at freshhempfoods.com and oneluckyduck.com.

Honey, Raw: You should be able to find raw honey at health food stores, or try raw food.com, oneluckyduck.com or reallyrawhoney.com.

Kaffir Lime Leaves: You can find these dried, at kalustyans.com, or fresh at import food.com.

Lecithin: Many health food stores carry lecithin, but be sure that it is made from non-GMO soy. You can find good quality lecithin at oneluckyduck.com or highvibe.com.

Maca: Peruvian maca is found in powder or capsule form at rawfood.com or onelucky duck.com.

Macadamia Nut Oil: We sell this in our shop in New York and on our website, and you can also find it at many upscale food retailers, or buy it directly at macnutoil.com.

Manna Bread: You can find the Nature's Path brand in the freezer section of most health food stores.

Maple Syrup Powder: Available at frontiercoop.com, shopnatural.com or sun organic.com.

Meyer Lemons: You can usually find organic Meyer lemons in season at any good health food store, or order online from Diamond Organics. If you are so inclined, you can actually grow your own indoor trees. See fourwindsgrowers.com for online ordering of baby Meyer lemon trees.

Microgreens: Greenmarkets are the best source, but at the restaurant, we also buy from Blue Moon Acres (215-794-3093). They are located in Buckingham, PA, and you can order by mail fresh, organic microgreens, and herbs.

Miso (Including Red Miso): South River Miso is our favorite and you can buy it at many health food stores, as well as directly from southrivermiso.com.

Nama Shoyu: You can generally find the Ohsawa brand of this unpasteurized soy sauce at any health food store, or online from rawfood.com.

Nutritional Yeast: This is often available in bulk bins at health food stores. To order organic nutritional yeast flakes online, the best source is frontiercoop.com. You can also find it at shopnatural.com.

Nuts, Raw Organic: Diamondorganics.com has a good selection, or try organicfruits andnuts.com.

Olive Oil and Other Oils: Rawfood.com and oneluckyduck.com sell good quality, cold-pressed organic olive oil. For good quality flaxseed oil and other seed oils, Flora is a very good brand: check florahealth.com for stores. Look for good quality nut oils at specialty shops.

Olives, Raw Organic: Available at rawfood.com and highvibe.com.

Pet Food, Raw: We have tried many varieties of raw pet food, and our favorite comes from amorepetfoods.com. It's organic and comes in individual packages so it's easy to use and our cats love it. Look for brands that use organic ingredients and do not include fillers such as grains. Another good source is auntjeni.com or grandads petfoods.com, although these may not be sold in individual portions. For the best treats your pet will love, try WildSide Salmon Freeze-Dried Cat (or Dog) Treats, available at catconnection.com.

Pistachios, Sicilian: Available at kalustyans.com.

Preserved Lemon Powder: Available at kalustyans.com.

Produce: Of course greenmarkets and local organic stores are the best sources, but if you are in a remote area, diamondorganics.com is a very good source for organic produce as well as many other organic foods and ingredients.

Salt: Celtic sea salt can be found at most health food stores, or you can buy it at celtic-seasalt.com. For Himalayan crystal salt go to transitionnutrition.com. We also carry both at oneluckyduck.com.

Sea Vegetables: At home we use Maine Coast Sea Vegetables very often, which you can find at most health food stores, or online at seaveg.com. You can also find untoasted nori and other seaweeds at shopnatural.com.

Spices: You should be able to find most of what you need at a local health food store, but you can also buy a wide variety of good quality bulk organic spices at frontier coop.com, including dried chili peppers.

Stevia: You can find both the liquid and powdered forms in the supplements section of most health food stores or at oneluckyduck.com.

Super Green Food: There are many brands of this powder available but the very best that we have come across are Pure Synergy and Nature's First Food and can be found at oneluckyduck.com, highvibe.com or rawfood.com.

Tamarind Pulp: The best kind to use comes in a block, sold as "seedless tamarind" at ethnicgrocer.com, or kalustyans.com.

Tocotrienols (TOCOS): Available at oneluckyduck.com or rawfood.com.

Truffles (Whole, and Black Truffle Paste): Gourmetfoodstore.com sells both. You can also order from S.O.S. Chefs in New York City (212-505-5813), where we buy ours for the restaurant.

Umeboshi Plum Paste: You can find the paste and the vinegar at most health food stores, or online at shopnatural.com.

Vanilla Beans: You can buy organic vanilla beans at most health food stores or at frontiercoop.com. They cost about $6.00 per bean, so you can also always substitute about 2 teaspoons of vanilla extract per $1/2$ vanilla bean.

Vanilla Extract: Nielsen-Massey Organic Madagascar Bourbon Pure Vanilla is the best quality organic vanilla to buy. The organic variety costs about 20 percent more than the equivalent inorganic vanilla from the same company. You can find it at cooking.com and oneluckyduck.com. You can also buy Frontier organic vanilla at frontiercoop.com, which sells for about 25 percent less on a per-ounce basis than the Nielsen-Massey organic variety. Most health food stores carry this brand as well.

Yacon Syrup: Available at oneluckyduck.com and rawfood.com.

Za'atar: Available at kalustyans.com (where they spell it "zaa'tar").

RECOMMENDED READING

Below is a brief list of some of our favorite (and inspiring!) resource books, all of which focus on raw foods (except for *Diet For a New America*, a very compelling, well-researched and eye-opening classic about healthy eating). These books and others that we find very valuable and informative on a variety of raw food and health related subjects are available at amazon.com and bookstores.

Conscious Eating (2nd edition) by Dr. Gabriel Cousens, M.D., North Atlantic Books, 2000.

Diet for a New America (reprint edition) by John Robbins, H. J. Kramer, 1998.

Eating for Beauty (3rd edition) by David Wolfe, Maul Brothers Publishing, 2003.

The Hippocrates Diet and Health Program by Ann Wigmore, Avery Publishing Group, 1984 (and any other book by Ann Wigmore).

LifeFood Recipe Book—Living on Life Force by Annie Padden Jubb and David Jubb, North Atlantic Books, 2003.

Living Cuisine by Renee Loux-Underkoffler, Avery Publishing Group, 2003.

Rainbow Green Live—Food Cuisine by Gabriel Cousens, M.D., North Atlantic Books, 2003.

The Sunfood Diet Success System (3rd edition) by David Wolfe, Maul Brothers Publishing, 2000.

ACKNOWLEDGMENTS
THANK YOU!!

Our foray into the world of raw foods was made possible by our good friend, **Robb Matzner**, who dragged us, reluctantly, to the meal that changed our lives. His wisdom and warmth continues to guide us today. At a time when we had more passion to open a restaurant than we knew what to do with, **Jeffrey Chodorow** allowed us to realize our dream. His knowledge, support (and stories) are a large part of our story. What would a raw restaurant be without a beautiful backyard garden? **Linda Chodorow** created one that is magical.

Doing business with friends is supposed to be difficult—this was not the case with our emotional restaurant builder, **Russell**

Muise. And he now has the glow. We are forever thankful to **JT McKay** for believing in us and helping us find our roadmap—and to **Terry Zarikian** whose belief in our vision helped give us this great opportunity.

In our new world, we were greeted by some of the brightest, most interesting people—their dedication helped give us the strength to embark on an entirely new path. **Denise Mari** (who has the clearest eyes of all) and **Doug Evans** created the forum for some of our first glimpses into this lifestyle. The writings and guidance of **David Jubb**, **Renee Underkoffler**, and **David Wolfe** continue to support and inspire us.

Our ever evolving restaurant is in the hands of some of the most talented professionals we have ever met—Chefs **Amanda Cohen**, **Glory Mongin** and Pastry Chef **Emily Cavelier** surprise us each day with an amazing level of dedication, creativity, and skill. We are also deeply grateful to have worked with **Debbie Lee**, **Valentin Studzinskiy**, and **Louisa Shafia**. Spreading the word about raw food must have been a real challenge—still, **Karine Bakhoum** and **Patricia Clough** did it with amazing grace. We are grateful for the warmth, dedication, and passion of every single person, past and present, that has helped make Pure Food and Wine so special, including **Gabriel Villa** and **Patrick Kenney**, who finally brought his enthusiasm for business and all things raw back to New York.

The opportunity to write this book, to express our vision, was an invaluable gift. **Judith Regan** made this possible. **Aliza Fogelson**'s grace and editing talents brought this book together and **Michelle Ishay**'s style and passion made it come alive. We thank **Charles Schiller** for his stunning photography, **Bette Blau** for her incredible eye and good taste, and finally, our collaborator, **Jen Karetnick**, for her wit, poetry, and good cyber-company during all the long hours.

Matthew would like to thank in particular...

My parents, **Robert** and **Shirley Kenney**, for helping me to see the beauty in nature at such a young age. Our special friend, supporter, adviser, and consultant **Glen Rosenberg** for always having our back. My warmest thanks are for **Sarma**. I greatly admire her professionalism, creative talent, and determination and have been blessed forever by the gift of her love.

Sarma would like to thank in particular...

My father, **John Melngailis**, for keeping me well fed with plenty of yummy fresh fruits and vegetables when I was little. My sweet mother, **Susan Jasse**, for teaching me to love and respect good food. My stepmother, **Michaele Weissman**, for eternal warmth and good advice. My stepfather, **Bob Jasse**, for always reminding me that you don't have to be a boy to have big balls. My sister, **Ilze**, and brother, **Noah**, for being such great allies in life. **Doug Evans** for opening my eyes one discouraging day to the fact that "It's all *good*." **Jesus Villafan**, just for being so good. **Rose Marie Swift**, for helping to show me (and the rest of the world) that makeup and lotion are food, too. And **Matthew**, for your patience, unconditional love, and collaboration in this crazy adventure that is our work and life. You are my angel.

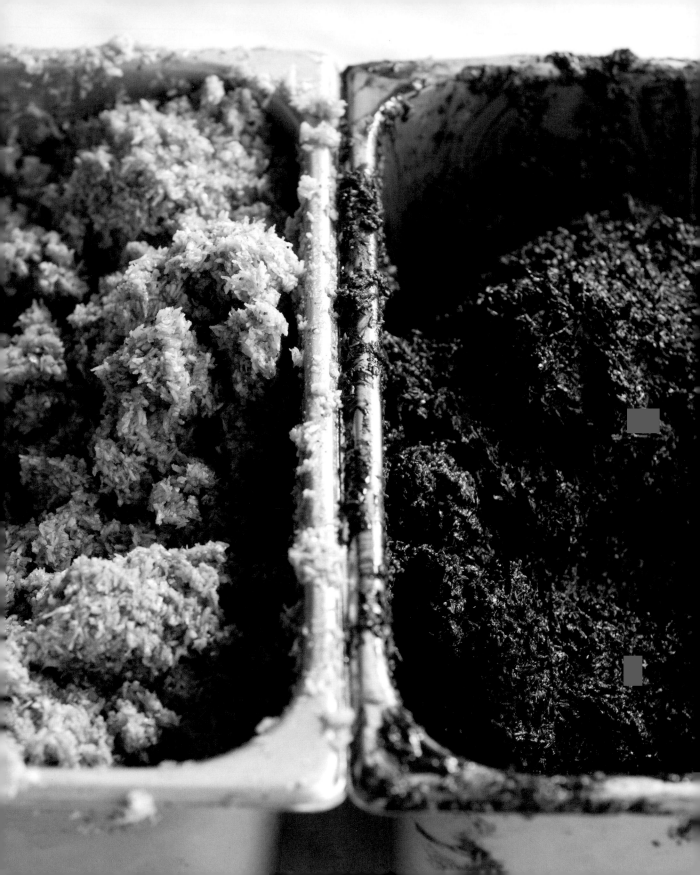

INDEX